W9-DFP-132

# THE
# ARTERIAL CIRCULATION

*Physical Principles and Clinical Applications*

---

## JOHN K-J. LI, PHD

*Department of Biomedical Engineering*
*Rutgers University, Piscataway, NJ*

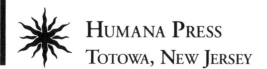

HUMANA PRESS
TOTOWA, NEW JERSEY

© 2000 Humana Press Inc.
999 Riverview Drive, Suite 208
Totowa, New Jersey 07512

For additional copies, pricing for bulk purchases, and/or information about other Humana titles, contact Humana at the above address or at any of the following numbers: Tel.: 973-256-1699; Fax: 973-256-8341; E-mail: humana@humanapr.com, or visit our Website: http://humanapress.com.

All rights reserved.

No part of this book may be reproduced, stored in a retrieval system, or transmitted in any form or by any means, electronic, mechanical, photocopying, microfilming, recording, or otherwise without written permission from the Publisher.

Due diligence has been taken by the publishers, editors, and author of this book to assure the accuracy of the information published and to describe generally accepted practices. The contributors herein have carefully checked to ensure that the drug selections and dosages set forth in this text are accurate and in accord with the standards accepted at the time of publication. Notwithstanding, as new research, changes in government regulations, and knowledge from clinical experience relating to drug therapy and drug reactions constantly occurs, the reader is advised to check the product information provided by the manufacturer of each drug for any change in dosages or for additional warnings and contraindications.

This is of utmost importance when the recommended drug herein is a new or infrequently used drug. It is the responsibility of the treating physician to determine dosages and treatment strategies for individual patients. Further, it is the responsibility of the health care provider to ascertain the Food and Drug Administration status of each drug or device used in their clinical practice. The publisher, editors, and authors are not responsible for errors or omissions or for any consequences from the application of the information presented in this book and make no warranty, express or implied, with respect to the contents in this publication.

All articles, comments, opinions, conclusions, or recommendations are those of the author(s), and do not necessarily reflect the views of the publisher.

Cover design by Patricia F. Cleary.

This publication is printed on acid-free paper.  ∞

ANSI Z39.48-1984 (American National Standards Institute) Permanence of Paper for Printed Library Materials).

**Photocopy Authorization Policy:**

Authorization to photocopy items for internal or personal use, or the internal or personal use of specific clients, is granted by Humana Press Inc., provided that the base fee of US $10.00 per copy, plus US $00.25 per page, is paid directly to the Copyright Clearance Center at 222 Rosewood Drive, Danvers, MA 01923. For those organizations that have been granted a photocopy license from the CCC, a separate system of payment has been arranged and is acceptable to Humana Press Inc. The fee code for users of the Transactional Reporting Service is: [0-89603-633-2/00 $10.00 + $00.25].

Printed in the United States of America.   10   9   8   7   6   5   4   3   2   1

ISBN 0-089603-633-2

*To my parents, Dr. George Tien-Fu Li, MD, and Yin-Chu Pan, RN,*
*for always being content with my accomplishments.*

*To my sons, Michael of Johns Hopkins,*
*and Christopher of Harvard, who have made me ever so proud.*

# PREFACE

After yet another decade of learning, experimenting, and investigating since my first book, *Arterial System Dynamics*, the many new medical breakthroughs and technological advances have inspired me to write this book to bridge the gap between basic research and clinical applications. The application of physical principles and quantitative approaches to the understanding of the arterial circulation and its interactions with the heart in normal and diseased conditions form the basis of *The Arterial Circulation*. Knowledge of the physiology and rheology of arteries, as well as all of their structural–functional correlates, is a necessary prerequisite to the proper hemodynamic interpretation of pressure–flow relations and the pulsatile transmission characteristics in different arteries. The natural coupling and interactions of the heart, the coronary circulation, and the arterial system necessitate analysis of alterations to global functioning. Modeling provides a tool for isolating and predicting parameter changes and is employed throughout the book. Experimental data are provided for model validations, and also for more realistic interpretations. Techniques and new methods for clinical hemodynamic measurement and diagnosis are included to help the reader understand the physical principles underlying such abnormal cardiovascular functions as hypertension, stenosis, and myocardial ischemia. The progressive changes in vascular properties during aging are also discussed. Modern approaches utilizing computer modeling and allomery are presented with selected examples, such as combined hypertension and aortic valve stenosis, and ventricular hypertrophy. The overall treatment is based on physical principles, with physiological relevance and clinical applications in mind. *The Arterial Circulation* is written for students, physiologists, biomedical engineers, pharmacologists, cardiologists, and other clinicians with a common interest in overall cardiovascular function.

Finally, I would like to thank all those who have contributed to the completion of this book.

*John K-J. Li, PHD*

# CONTENTS

# ABOUT THE AUTHOR

Dr. Li is a Professor II (distinguished) and Director of Cardiovascular Research in the Department of Biomedical Engineering at Rutgers, The State University, Piscataway, NJ. He is a Fellow of the American College of Cardiology, a Fellow of the American College of Angiology, and a Fellow of the American Institute of Medical and Biological Engineering.

# 1 INTRODUCTION

## 1.1. Historical View of Arterial Circulation

The heart and the arterial system are such close functional complements that the circulatory system cannot be effectively described by either one alone. Only by virtue of the distributing arterial trees can oxygen, humoral agents, and nutrients be transported to the vital parts of the body, while the heart provides the necessary energy.

The observation that humans must inspire air to sustain life led ancient scientists and philosophers to toy with the idea that arteries contained air rather than blood. This notion was originally attributed to Erasistratus in the third century BC, following the teaching of Aristotle. That arteries contract and relax had been known in Aristotle's time. Galen later (130–200 AD) described the ebb and flow of blood in arteries, which, though it lasted for centuries, was grossly inaccurate. Additionally, in the Galenic view, blood was passed from the right side of the heart to the left side through pores, which was later shown to be incorrect, because they do not exist within the interventricular septum. This open-circuit interpretation does not accurately describe the circulation of blood. Galileo (1564–1642) in his *Dialogue of the Two Sciences*, which appeared in 1637, suggested the circulation of blood in a closed system. Today, the idea of the circulation of blood is credited to William Harvey (1578–1657), a contemporary of Galileo, in his now famous *De Motu Cordis and De Circulatione Sanguinis* (1628). He described in his *Anatomical Exercises* explained that "blood does continually passes through the heart" and that "blood flows continually out the arteries and into the veins." His work was completed before Malphighi, who worked with the aid of a microscope, and discovered the capillaries in 1661, which linked the arterial circulation to the venous circulation. Harvey's work indicated the pulsatile nature of blood as a consequence of intermittent inflow, during roughly one-third of the heart cycle, now known as systole, in combination with essentially steady outflow through the periphery during the remaining cardiac period, the diastole.

Fascinated by the anatomic structure of the vascular tree, Leonardo da Vinci (1452–1519) made many detailed drawings of the constituent parts of the circulatory system. He apparently already knew that both contrac-

From: *Arterial Circulation: Physical Principles and Clinical Applications*
By: J. K-J. Li © Humana Press Inc., Totowa, NJ

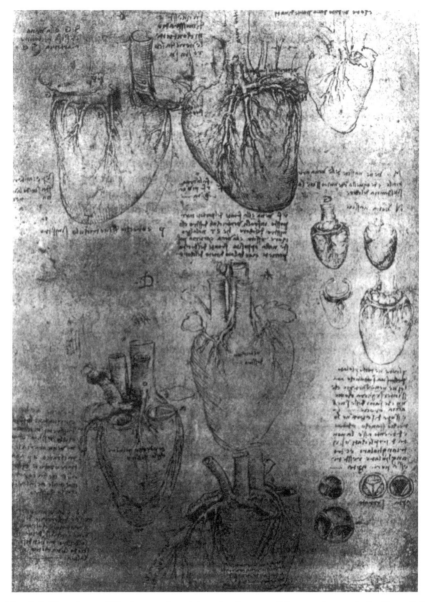

Fig. 1-1. Drawings of the human heart, heart valves, and the great vessels by the artist Leonardo da Vinci. Shape and size are shown in good geometric proportions. Coronary arteries and their major branches, as well as leaflets of the valves are well illustrated.

tion and resting periods are necessary for the heart to function with a normal rhythm. His anatomic drawings of the heart and the perfusing arteries are amazingly accurate: Figure 1-1 illustrates one such drawing, in

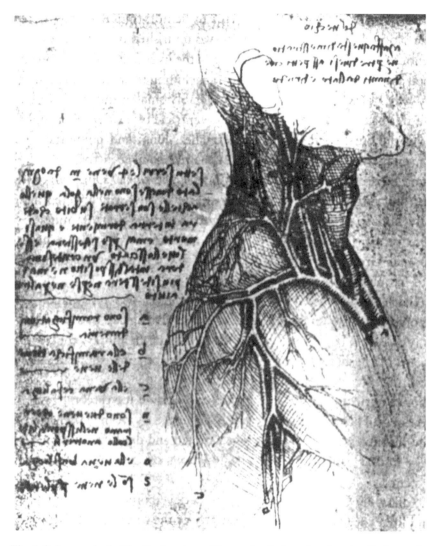

Fig. 1-2. Leonardo da Vinci's drawing of the neck arteries, showing detailed vascular branching morphology. Branching angles and generations are carefully drawn.

which the heart and the great vessels are clearly seen, together with the main, anterior descending and circumflex coronary arteries and their major branches. Several drawings of the heart valves are also shown, demonstrating how well the leaflets are arranged when the valves are closed. He has also provided the detailed anatomic drawing of the neck arteries in humans with its branching morphology clearly shown, including the subclavian, carotid, and brachial arteries (Fig. 1-2). Both the length and angle of branching arteries are highly accurate. His annotations with these drawings are depicted in many of the historical notes of the circulation. Vesalius (1514–1564), an anatomist, later provided a detailed drawing of the entire human vascular tree.

The beating of the heart generates pressure and flow pulsations. Ancient Chinese practitioners customarily felt palpable wrist artery (radial artery) pulsations as a means of diagnosing the cardiac state of their patients. In this approach, the practitioners were able to obtain both the strength of the pulsation, to infer the vigor of contraction of the heart, and the interval duration of the pulses, and hence heart rate. This may indicate that the importance of the rate–pressure product, now a popular clinical index of myocardial oxygen consumption, was considered pertinent even at that time. The supply and demand of oxygenation, as well as its proper utilization in terms of energy balance, or ying-yang, is central to achieving body harmony. Thus, the suggestion of an intrinsic transfer of energy (Chi) generated by the heart to the peripheral arteries may have been known since antiquity, although the theoretical foundation was not established until much later.

The measurements of the magnitudes of blood pressure (BP) and flow took considerably longer than the interpretation of the circulatory function. In 1733, Stephan Hales had incidentally already registered the magnitude of the BP level about which blood oscillates. His initial measurement of BP with a glass tube in a horse has been well illustrated in many publications (Fig. 1-3). Thus, the magnitude of the mean arterial pressure and the amplitude of oscillation, or the pulse pressure (PP), were already known at that time. Hales' measurements, accounted in his *Haemastaticks*, however, did not induce recognition of the great importance of the magnitudes of BP on cardiac function for many decades. Now, we know how the increased magnitudes of mean BP and PP are major contributors to hypertension and many forms of cardiovascular diseases.

The shape of the pressure pulse, however, became known only in the nineteenth century, when Ludwig (1847) invented the kymograph, which inscribed blood pressure waveforms. His instrument provided information on BP within a single beat which was a truly a technological advance, although its accuracy was not comparable to present-day instruments. Blood pressure recording with sphygmographs by Marey and his contemporary Mahomed (1872) led to the clinical assessment of arterial diseases, such as hypertension. Chaveau and Marey (1863) also recorded cardiac chamber pressures, and both later measured blood flow with an instrument they developed, now known as the bristle flowmeter.

Modern development of BP and blood flow waveforms came with the inventions of the fluid-filled catheter–manometer system (Li et al., 1976)

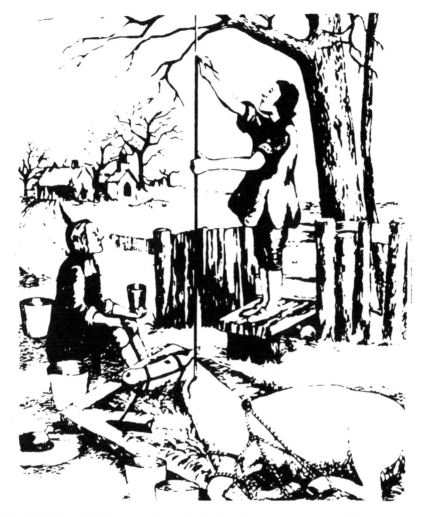

Fig. 1-3. Hales (1733) apparently made the first direct measurement of the magnitude of the BP level about which blood oscillates. His initial measurement of BP with a glass tube in a horse neck artery is illustrated.

and the electromagnetic flowmeter. The simultaneous measurements of BP and flow have led to the considerable advancement of the studies of blood flow or hemodynamics. The catheter was introduced in humans by Forssmann (1929) and later advanced for catheterization of right heart for pressure measurement by Cournand and Range (1941). The flowmeter was introduced by Kolin (1936) and was subsequently modified by Franklin et al. (1961). Cournand and Forssmann shared the Nobel prize with Richards for medicine in 1956 for the invention and advancement of modern day catheterization for visualization of BP waveforms in various anatomical sites throughout the circulation.

Apart from his interest in the arterial circulation, Hales (1733) also measured ventricular volumes in several species of mammals (*see* Chapter 7). He concluded that in order for the arteries to accept the large amount of ejected blood, or the stroke volume, the arteries must behave like a temporary storage reservoir. Because the size of the aorta is considerably smaller than that of the ventricle, the receiving aorta must be elastic, in order to perform the function of a reservoir. This interpretation of the reservoir function of arteries, introduced by this English Fellow of the Royal Society, became known as the windkessel theory, which was vigorously pursued over a century later by a German physician, Otto Frank (1899). The emphasis on the storage properties of the arteries, which were modeled by Frank as a single elastic tube (*see* Fig. 3-1) implied that all pressure fluctuations in the arterial tree should occur synchronously, i.e., the BP pulse should propagate with infinite velocity. The peripheral vessels, on the other hand were assumed rigid as stiff tubes, which gave rise to the lumped compliance-resistance model of the arterial circulation. This windkessel model lacks the description of the propagation characteristics of the pressure pulse.

Finite velocity of blood pressure pulse propagation in a blood vessel was considered over two centuries ago by Euler (1775), who attempted to develop a formula for its calculation. The well-known physicist Thomas Young (1816), and also the Weber brothers (1866), apparently solved the propagation velocity in an elastic tube (Noordergraaf, 1969). Incorporating the elastic properties and geometry of the blood vessel, Moens (1878) and Korteweg (1878) separately developed what is now known as the Moens-Korteweg formula for the pulse wave velocity (PWV):

$$c_0 = \sqrt{Eh/2r\rho} \qquad (1\text{-}1)$$

where E, is, appropriately at the time, defined as the Young's modulus of elasticity of the blood vessel, $h$ and $r$ are the wall thickness and inner radius of the uniform cylindrical vessel (Fig. 1-4), respectively, and $\rho$ is the density of blood. Pulse propagation velocity is seen to be related to the mechanical and geometrical properties of the blood vessel.

## *1.2. Recent Developments*

Much of the modern development of the theory related to the transmission of blood pressure pulse waveform has been motivated by the shortcomings of the windkessel theory formulated by Frank. Witzig's (1914) little known doctoral dissertation had already led to the mathematical formulation of blood flow through elastic tubes. Womersley's (1957) theory

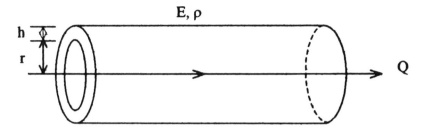

Fig. 1-4. Uniform cylindrical vessel representation of the blood vessel with inner radius, $r$, and wall thickness, $h$. Young's modulus of elasticity of the blood vessel wall, E, and the density of blood, $\rho$, are also shown.

of oscillating flow in an elastic tube was extensively used in mathematical modeling of the arteries. McDonald's *Blood Flow in Arteries* (1960) was the first text that dealt exclusively with the subject; now in its fourth edition, it familiarized readers with theoretical development and experimental measurements. Modeling efforts have been extensively reviewed by Noordergraaf (1969,1978) and Li (1987). These texts also provided experimental measurement methods and quantitative approaches to the assessments of the state of the arterial circulation.

In the application to clinical situations, Wiggers (1928) extensively studied the morphology of blood pressure waveforms and their relations to varied diseased conditions. This concept was recently revisited by others following similar fundamental paths of descriptions of the features of the arterial pulse in disease diagnosis. New groups of drugs that act differently from vasodilators, β-adrenergic blockers, calcium channel blockers, and angiotensin-converting enzyme inhibitors now afford locally targeted vascular drug delivery, as well as gene therapy. They improve vascular perfusion and in the treatment of diseases.

The extensive use of the electrical transmission line analogy to blood flow beginning in the 1950s, has enabled the impedance concept to be applied to the arterial circulation. Impedance can be considered as complex resistance whose value changes with frequency; unlike resistance, whose value is normally constant and independent of frequency. Thus, the arterial circulation can no longer be viewed as resistance vessels, but are compliant with elastic properties that vary with frequency. The classical elastic description of blood vessels has been modified to include viscosity of the blood and the arterial wall. Viscosity causes energy dissipation. Arteries by nature are viscoelastic rather than purely elastic. Regarding Chi, or energy considerations, the amount of work that the heart must generate during each beat has generated considerable attention. This work included the steady energy dissipation through peripheral resistance vessels in different parts of the body, as well as energy required to overcome pulsations, which persist even in the microcirculation.

Modeling has been a necessary path in the understanding of circulatory system properties. It is difficult to experimentally or clinically measure simultaneous pressure and flow at certain anatomical sites; modeling thus provides a solution in predicting pressure and flow at inaccessible sites and the interpretation of features of the waveforms, when looking at the complex multibranching network of the vascular tree. This has been well-illustrated by many texts, such as those by McDonald (1960), Wetterer and Kenner (1968), Noordergraaf (1978), and Li (1987,1996). Linear theories have been utilized by numerous investigators. Usefulness of linear theories has recently been discussed (Li et al., 1981,1984). Linearity assumes superposition and periodicity. However, nonlinearities do exist, such as the nonlinear change of arterial compliance with blood pressure levels and the appearance of flow turbulence. Both linear and nonlinear theories of pulse wave transmission and modeling of the arterial system require experimental verification. This latter was met by the advancement in instrumentation for pressure, flow, and dimension measurements.

Clinical applications of modern developments in hemodynamics have initiated both invasive and noninvasive measurements, including vascular imaging. Assessments of vascular hypertrophy, hypertension, and atherosclerosis have all utilized the quantification of parameters derived from hemodynamic theories and models. Some of these parameters are wave reflections, arterial compliance changes, and vascular stiffness, just to name a few.

### 1.3. Book Content

This book is centered on the arterial circulation. The book was written utilizing fundamental physical principles to establish hemodynamic methods, in order to provide a basis for clinical measurement and interpretation of the hemodynamic conditions of patients. It deals with the structural and functional aspects of the arterial system, theories and experiments on the transmission characteristics of pressure and flow pulsations, with energy considerations, and the use of modern instrumentation for hemodynamic measurements for quantitative assessment of the arterial system, with an emphasis on the clinical applications.

In Chapter 2, the anatomical aspects of the arterial tree are first illustrated. These include the major branches of human and dog arteries, since hemodynamic experimental data are collected most commonly in these two mammalian species. Nonuniformities in geometry and elastic properties are examined. Geometric nonuniformities include tapering and vascular branching; nonuniformities in elasticity include the content and organization of the arterial wall. Constituent structural components of the arterial wall are examined in rheological terms, particularly, the physical properties of elastin, collagen, and smooth muscle. Differences in their mechanical properties in large and small arteries are examined and their collective contributions to the arterial wall function are analyzed. The arterial wall does not merely behave as an elastic vessel, therefore viscoelastic behavior becomes important. In this context, the viscous and elastic behavior of the composite, i.e., the arterial wall, is discussed, including the characteristics of a viscoelastic material, i.e., creep phenomenon, stress relaxation, and hysteresis.

Chapter 3 deals with blood pressure and flow pulse wave transmission characteristics in terms of simplified mathematical description and fundamental modeling principles. The classic description of the windkessel model of the arterial system is first introduced. The windkessel is the most used lumped model of the arterial system in the clinical setting, therefore, its analysis is elaborated in terms of total arterial system compliance and peripheral resistance. Extension of this model to more sophisticated later models includes those that vary from a linear rigid tube model to a freely moving or constrained thin- or thick-walled, viscoelastic tube model. Some of these utilize Navier-Stokes equations describing fluid motion, Navier equations describing wall movement, and the equation of continuity describing incompressibility of blood. Experimental deviations from linear models are compared to nonlinear theories, in order to identify the regimes of nonlinearities.

Distributed models provide more precise descriptions of the pressure and flow behavior under varied conditions. However, they are generally complex and time-consuming in identifying individual parameters, and less useful in daily clinical settings. Reduced models that are useful for practical and clinical applications are discussed. Relative advantages of electrical analogs are also compared, including the model that describes an isolated arterial segment, such as the descending thoracic aorta or relatively uniform arteries, such as the femoral and the carotid artery. A recently introduced model to analyze arterial wall behavior subject to varying pressure amplitudes, in terms of pressure-dependent compliance, is elaborated. This helps to explain the cyclical stress placed on the arterial wall and how the arterial wall adjusts to rapidly changing pressure amplitudes.

Once models of the arterial system have been developed, it is necessary to verify their validity and limitations. Such verifications often depend critically on the specific design of experiments for measuring relevant hemodynamic parameters. For all practical purposes, these are pressure, flow, velocity, and vessel dimensions.

Pulsatile pressure and flow and their transmission characteristics are the central points of Chapter 4, in which the peculiarities and features associated with pressure and flow waveforms, measured in their respective anatomical sites, are explained. How the vascular beds present as load impeding blood flow is quantitatively described in terms of the vascular impedance concept. Impedance, unlike resistance, which remains constant, is complex, as its magnitude changes with frequency. Its usefulness is in its ability to include alterations in compliance, resistance, and inertance. This impedance concept provides a useful description of the changing arterial tree and individual vascular bed behavior.

How efficiently the pressure pulse transmits depends on the propagation and reflection characteristics through different arteries and vascular branching junctions. PWV, a popularly used index to describe vascular stiffness, is dependent on the geometric and elastic properties of the local arterial wall. Its measurement is therefore elaborated.

With differing vascular impedances, wave reflections arise, because of the mismatching in impedances. The large peripheral resistances in the arterioles are the principal sites contributing to reflections. Increased wave reflection increases BP amplitude, and thus decreases flow. This reduces the pulse transmission efficiency for the propagating pulse. Pulse propagation and reflections in the arterial system are also analyzed in Chapter 4. Pulse transmission through vascular branching junctions are dictated by local blood vessel properties. For the forward-traveling wave, it is practically impedance-matched at vascular junctions, resulting in optimal transmission. The backward-traveling wave, toward the heart, is greatly attenuated at the vascular branching. Thus, the design of the arterial tree facilitates pulse transmission to vascular beds. These aspects are discussed in detail for their importance in both basic and clinical situations. Pulse pressure and flow remain pulsatile even in the microcirculation, althought at a much-reduced amplitude. The pulsatility facilitates capillary exchanges.

Clinically useful methods and instruments for invasive and noninvasive determination of BP, flow, cardiac output, and vessel dimensions are presented in Chapter 5, begining with the auscultatory method, the use of sphygmomanometer cuff method, oscillometric method, and extending to the modern use of tonometry. These are commonly used and noninvasive methods. Clinical catheterization laboratories are mostly equipped with catheter-manometer systems for invasive blood pressure waveform and thermodilution measurements. The frequency response and usefulness of catheter-based monitoring is elaborated. Principles of thermodilution and its clinical utilization are demonstrated.

BF measurement has generally been limited to the electromagnetic flowmeter in the experimental setting, and to the Doppler ultrasonic method for blood velocity measurement in the clinical setting. The former is mostly invasive; the latter is mostly noninvasive. Combination of Doppler velocity measurement and vascular imaging has been popular with the advent of Doppler echocardiography and intravascular imaging devices.

Chapter 6 deals with the performance of the heart and the arterial circulation, the important aspect of their coupling, and dynamic beat-to-beat interaction. Ventricular and arterial elastances under steady-state conditions are described, and their usefulness and limitations are addressed. The concept of dynamic arterial elastance, in terms of dynamic arterial compliance and dynamic interaction of the heart and the arterial system within a single heartbeat, are also discussed. For instance, the improvement of arterial compliance and reduction of wave reflection has been one of the central treatment strategies involving hypertensive patients.

Coronary arterial circulation, which perfuses the heart, is an important aspect of arterial circulation, and its pressure-flow characteristics and modeling aspect in terms of beat-to-beat myocardial function, is explained. The obvious clinical significance is illustrated with examples such as coronary arterial stenosis and myocardial ischemia.

Some of the newer aspects in the analysis and treatment strategies of hypertension and cardiac hypertrophy, based on understanding of the arterial system, are discussed in Chapter 7. These include the use of critical hemodynamic parameters, such as arterial compliance and wave reflection in the assessment of the severity and in the evaluation of therapeutical effectiveness. From this perspective, the close association of aging and hypertension is analyzed. Understanding the structural and functional significance of cardiovascular changes associated with aging has become an important aspect of clinical cardiology.

Analysis of the double-loaded ventricle, which faces both aortic valve stenosis and increased arterial system load, is also presented. This aspect demonstrates the use of modeling in modern clinical diagnosis and its potential use in treatment strategy.

Experiments that have been designed to study arterial dynamics are mostly performed in animals. It is thus important to investigate the similarity of the cardiovascular system across mammalian species. The use of allometry, dimensional analysis, and the Π-theorem of Buckingham are also introduced in Chapter 7. Application of these to established hemodynamic similarity principles are systematically illustrated, and their limitations are discussed. Whether similarity reflects optimality, in terms of structure-function design features, is elucidated, as well as the diagnostic applications of the similarity principles. Diagnostic allometry may present itself as the newest class of methodology in the treatment of patients.

# REFERENCES

Chaveau, A. and Marey, E. Appareils et experiences cardiographiques. Demonstration nouvelle de mechanisms des mouvements du coeur par l'emploi des instruments enregistreurs a indications continues. *Mem. Acad. Med.* 26:268, 1863.

Courand, A. and Ranges, H. A. Catheterization of the right auricle in man. *Proc. Soc. Exp. Biol. Med.* 46:462–466, 1941.

Euler, L. *Principes generaux du mouvement des fluides.* History Academy, Berlin, 1775.

Fich, S. and Li, J. K.-J. Aorto-ventricular dynamics: theories, experiments, and instrumentation. *CRC Crit. Rev. Biomed. Eng.* 9:245–285, 1983.

Forssmann, W. Die Sondierung des rechten Herzens. *Klin. Wochschr.* 8:2085, 1929.

Frank, O. Die Grundform des arteriellen Pulses. *Z. Biol.* 37:483–526, 1899.

Franklin, D. L., Schlegel, W., and Rushmer, R. F. Blood flow measured by Doppler frequency shift back-scattered ultrasound. *Science* 134:564–565, 1961.

Galilei, G. *Dialogues Concerning Two New Sciences.* 1637. Translated version (Crew, H. and DeSalvio, A.), Macmillan, New York, 1914.

Hales, S. *Statical Essays Containing Haemostaticks.* London, 1733.

Harvey, W. *De Motu Cordis* and *De Circulatione Sanquinis.* London, 1628.

Kolin, A. Electromagnetic flowmeter. The principle of the method and its application to blood flow measurement. *Proc. Soc. Exp. Biol. Med.* 35:53–56, 1936.

Korteweg, D. J. Uber die Fortpflanzungsgeschwindigkeit des Schalles in elastischen Rohren. *Ann. Phys. Chem.* 5:525–537, 1878.

Li, J. K-J., Van Brummelen, A. G. W., and Noordergraaf, A. Fluid-filled blood pressure measurement systems. *J. Appl. Physiol.* 40:839–843, 1976.

Li, J. K-J., Melbin, J., Riffle, R. A., and Noordergraaf, A. Pulses wave propagation. *Circ. Res.* 49:442–452, 1981.

Li, J. K-J., Melbin, J., and Noordergraaf, A. Directional disparity of pulse wave reflections in dog arteries. *Am. J. Physiol.* 247:H95–H99, 1984.

Li, J. K-J. *Arterial System Dynamics.* New York University Press, New York, 1987.

Li, J. K-J. *Comparative Cardiovascular Dynamics of Mammals.* CRC Press, New York, 1996.

Mahomed, F. A. Physiology and clinical use of the sphygmograph. *Med. Times Gaz.* 1:62, 1872.

McDonald, D. A. *Blood Flow in Arteries.* Arnold, London, 1960.

Moens, A. I. *Die Pulskurve.* Leiden, 1878.

Nichols W. W. and O'Rourke, M. F. *McDonald's Blood Flow in Arteries*, 4th ed., Arnold, London, 1998.

Noordergraaf, A. Hemodynamics. In: Schwan, H. P., ed., *Biological Engineering.* McGraw-Hill, New York, 1969.

Noordergraaf, A. *Circulatory System Dynamics.* Academic , New York, 1978.

Weber, E. H. Uber die Anwendung der Welienlehre auf die Lehre vom Kreislaufe des Blutes und ins Besondere auf die Pulsiehre. *Ber. Math. Physik, Cl. Konigl. Sachs. Ges. Wiss. 1850.*

Wiggers, C. J. *Pressure Pulse in the Cardiovascular System.* Longmans, London, 1928.

Wetterer, E. and Kenner, T. *Grundlagen der Dynamik des Arterienpulses.* Springer-Verlag, Berlin, 1968.

Womersley, J. R. Mathematical analysis of the arterial circulation in a state of oscillatory motion. *WADC Tech. Rep.* WADC-TR56-614, 1957.

Young T. Hydraulic investigations, subservient to an intended Croonian Lecture on the motion of the blood. *Philosoph. Trans.* 98:164-180, 1808.

Young T. On the functions of the heart and arteries (The Croonian Lecture). *Phil. Trans.* 99:1–31, 1809.

# 2 Physiology and Rheology of Arteries

## 2.1. Anatomical and Structural Organization

Anatomical descriptions of the human and other mammalian arterial trees can be found in many textbooks. For the purpose of illustrating the blood perfusion and pressure pulse transmission path, the major branches of the arterial tree are shown in Fig. 2-1. There are considerable similarities among the corresponding anatomical sites of the arterial circulation in mammals (Li, 1996). The root of the aorta begins immediately at the aortic valve. The outlet of the aortic valve sits in the ascending aorta, which has the largest diameter of the aorta. The first branches off the aorta are the left and right main coronary arteries. The aortic arch junction is formed by the ascending aorta, the brachiocephalic artery, the left subclavian artery, and the descending thoracic aorta.

Numerous branches come off the descending aorta at right angles, e.g., the renal arteries, which perfuse the kidneys. The distal end of the descending aorta is the abdominal aorta, which forms the aortoiliac junction, with left and right iliac arteries and its continuation. In the human, the junction is a bifurcation. The femoral artery, a well-known peripheral artery, because of its accessibility, continues from the iliac artery. These are the arteries perfusing the upper thighs, the tibial arteries perfuse the lower legs. The aorta has, comparatively, the greatest geometric taper, with its diameter decreasing with increasing distance away from the ventricle. The common carotid arteries are the longest, relatively uniform vessels, with the least geometrical tapering. The brachial arteries perfusing the upper arms lead to distal radial arteries. Both brachial and radial arteries are the most common sites for noninvasive blood pressure (BP) monitoring.

The arterial system is a tapered branching system. Changes in lumen size are often associated with branching and appropriate tapering. In the normal arterial system, the branched daughter vessels are always narrower than the mother vessel, but with slightly larger total cross-sectional areas. This means that the branching area ratio, or the ratio of the total cross-sectional area of the daughter vessels to that of the mother vessel, is slightly greater than 1. This has significance in terms of pulsatile energy transmission, which is discussed in Chapter 4, under pulse wave reflections (Subheading 4.4.).

From: *Arterial Circulation: Physical Principles and Clinical Applications*
By: J. K-J. Li © Humana Press Inc., Totowa, NJ

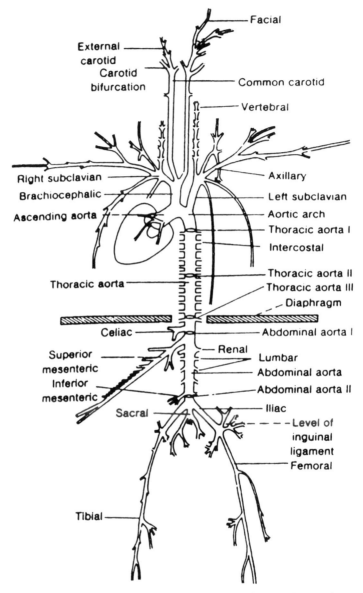

Fig. 2-1. Schematic representation of the arterial tree of a dog. Anatomic structures reveal geometric tapering and branching characteristics of the arterial system. Adapted with permission from McDonald (1974).

Arterial diameters and lumen areas of the vascular tree can be determined from postmortem cast or angioradiography. Arteries in man and in dog retract some 25–40% when removed (Bergel, 1961; Learoyd and Tay-

Table 2-1
Dimensions of Arteries in Dogs

| Artery | Radius (cm) | Area ($cm^2$) | Radius | Area | Radius | Area |
|---|---|---|---|---|---|---|
| Asc. aorta | 1.01 | 3.21 | 0.75 | 1.77 | 0.73 | 1.77 |
| Thor. A I | 0.82 | 2.11 | 0.55 | 0.95 | 0.48 | 0.78 |
| Thor. A II | 0.66 | 1.38 | 0.48 | 0.72 | 0.40 | 0.52 |
| Thor. A III | 0.61 | 1.19 | 0.45 | 0.64 | 0.39 | 0.51 |
| Abd. A I | 0.45 | 0.64 | 0.40 | 0.50 | 0.40 | 0.52 |
| Abd. A II | 0.44 | 0.60 | 0.35 | 0.38 | 0.35 | 0.39 |
| Brach. ceph. | 0.53 | 0.88 | 0.40 | 0.50 | 0.38 | 0.49 |
| L. Subcl. | 0.44 | 0.60 | 0.35 | 0.38 | 0.35 | 0.41 |
| Coeliac | 0.29 | 0.27 | 0.23 | 0.17 | 0.25 | 0.21 |
| Sup. mes. | 0.34 | 0.35 | 0.23 | 0.17 | 0.23 | 0.18 |
| Renal (2) | 0.19 | 0.12 | 0.15 | 0.07 | 0.19 | 0.12 |
| Iliac (2) | 0.23 | 0.17 | 0.24 | 0.18 | 0.23 | 0.13 |
| Sacral | 0.23 | 0.17 | 0.20 | 0.13 | 0.18 | 0.10 |
| Int. cost. (20) | 0.09 | 0.029 | 0.06 | 0.01 | 0.06 | 0.01 |
| Inf. mes. | – | – | 0.10 | 0.03 | 0.12 | 0.05 |
| Lumbar (8) | – | – | 0.10 | 0.03 | 0.08 | 0.02 |
| Comm. carot. | – | – | 0.20 | 0.13 | 0.25 | 0.20 |
| Vertebral (2) | – | – | 0.12 | 0.05 | – | – |
| R. subcl. | – | – | 0.28 | 0.25 | – | – |
| Axillary | – | – | 0.20 | 0.13 | – | – |
| Femoral | – | – | 0.15 | 0.07 | – | – |

Adapted with permission from McDonald (1974).

lor, 1966). It is therefore necessary that in vivo lengths are restored and that corresponding pressures are given. Under normal conditions, a higher distending pressure leads to a greater lumen diameter. Table 2-1 illustrates some arterial vessel dimensions (McDonald, 1974). The corresponding dimensions in humans have been provided, e.g., by Westerhof et al. (1969), for constructing the analog model of the human systemic arterial tree.

There are several branching junctions before the pulse reaches the vascular beds. In relation to this, the number of generations of blood vessels are given by Green (1950) and Iberall (1967).

Experimental data by Li (1978,1987) gives typical values of internal diameters in a 20-kg dog: ascending aorta, 15 mm; abdominal aorta, 8 mm; femoral artery, 3 mm; small artery, 0. 1 mm. These values reveal an appreciable geometric taper in the aorta from the root to the aortoiliac junction, which together with branching, contributes to the geometric nonuniformity observed throughout the arterial system.

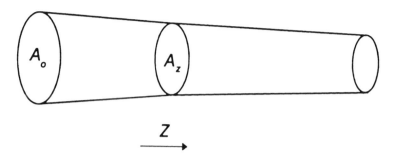

$$A(z) = A_o e^{-K_o Z}$$

Fig. 2-2. Schematic diagram illustrating a blood vessel with geometric taper. The vessel diameter narrows with increasing distance ($z$) away from the origin. Geometric taper, an exponential function of distance, is normally calculated from the change in cross-sectional areas ($A$), as shown.

The term "geometrical taper" is appropriate when applied to a single continuous conduit, such as the aorta. The area change of the aortic crosssection is close to an exponential form, (Fig. 2-2) and can be expressed as

$$A(z) = A(0) \exp(-kz/r) \qquad (2\text{-}1)$$

where $z$ = distance in the longitudinal axial direction along the vessel; $r$ = vessel lumen radius in cm; k = taper factor, dimensionless; $A(0)$ = the cross-sectional area at the entrance of the vessel in $cm^2$; and $A(z)$ = the cross-sectional at distance $z$ along the vessel in $cm^2$

The vessel area is calculated, assuming a circular cross-section,

$$A = \pi r^2 \qquad (2\text{-}2)$$

The taper factor, $k$, can be readily obtained as

$$k = \frac{r}{z} \ln \frac{A(o)}{A(z)} \qquad (2\text{-}3)$$

As an example, suppose the ascending aorta diameter for a 70-kg man is 3 cm and the terminal abdominal aorta diameter is 1.3 cm and the length of the aorta is 46 cm, then the taper factor for the aorta is

$$k = 0.024 \qquad (2\text{-}4)$$

Van der Werff (1974) reported a value of $k = 0.0367$ for a 30-kg dog. Ling et al. (1968) reported $k = 0.0328$ for a 22.1-kg dog. The calculated value from the above 20-kg dog is 0.0314 (Li, 1987). These values are not significantly different.

Table 2-2
**External Diameters and Taper Factors**

|  | d (cm) | ko (cm) |
|---|---|---|
| Abdominal aorta | 0.777 | $0.027 \pm 0.007$ |
| Iliac artery | 0.413 | $0.021 \pm 0.005$ |
| Femoral artery | 0.342 | $0.018 \pm 0.007$ |
| Carotid artery | 0.378 | $0.008 \pm 0.004$ |

Geometric taper factor can change substantially during varied vasoactive conditions and in disease conditions. When vasoactive drugs are administered, which have differential effects on large and small arteries, changes in taper factors from normal can be quite pronounced.

Alternative formula to calculate taper factor per unit length (Li, 1987), or $ko$, is shown below:

$$A(z) = A(0)e^{-koz} \tag{2-5}$$

The reported values of $ko$ obtained for the abdominal aorta and the iliac, femoral, and carotid arteries are shown in Table 2-2. These are measured in vivo, at a mean arterial pressure of about 90 mmHg. The average body weight of dogs used is about 20 kg. It is obvious from these data that the taper factor is smaller for smaller vessels. Carotid arteries have the least taper, and they are thus the best approximation to a geometrically uniform cylindrical vessel.

Area ratios calculated for vascular branching junctions were about 1.08 at the aortic arch and 1.05 at the aortoiliac junction (Li et al., 1984). These values are slightly larger than 1.0; the consequence of these results is discussed in Subheading 4.4.

In the broadest sense, the arterial wall (Fig. 2-3) consists of elastin, collagen, and smooth muscle embedded in a mucopolysaccharide ground substance. A cross-section reveals the tunica intima, which is the innermost layer, consisting of a thin layer (0.5–1 μm) of endothelial cells, connective tissue, and basement membrane. The next layer is the thick tunica media, separated from the intima by a prominent layer of elastic tissue: the internal lamina. The media contains elastin, smooth muscle, and collagen. The difference in their composition divides arteries into elastic and muscular vessels.

The relative content of these in different vessels is shown in Fig. 2-4. All vessels, including the capillary, have endothelium. The capillary does not have smooth muscle content, and has only a single layer of endothelial cells. The outermost layer is the adventitia, which is made up mostly of stiff collagenous fibers.

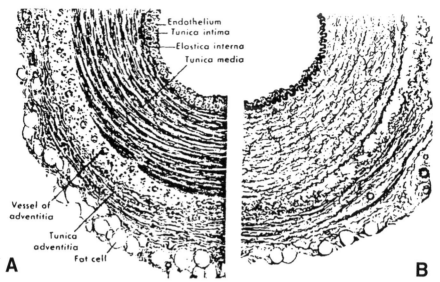

Fig. 2-3. Cross sections of a human artery reveal three distinctive layers: the innermost tunica intima, the thick tunica media, and the outermost adventitia. **(A)** Stained with hematoxin and eosin. **(B)** Stained with orcein. Adapted with permission from Bloom and Fawcett (1975).

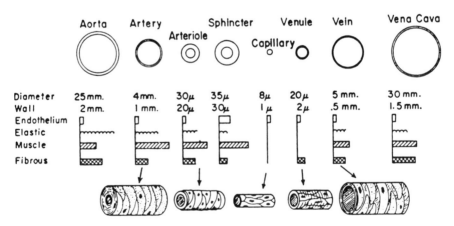

Fig. 2-4. Relative contents of endothelium, elastic and fibrous tissues, and smooth muscle in different vessels. Large arteries have more elastic and fibrous tissues while smaller arteries have more smooth muscle in the tunica media. Adapted with permission from Rushmer (1972).

Elastic laminae are concentrically distributed, and attached by smooth muscle cells and connective tissue. Longitudinally, we find that the number of elastic laminae decreases with increasing distance from the aorta, but the amount of smooth muscle increases, and the relative wall thickness increases. Thus, the wall thickness to radius ratio, or h/r is increased. The net stiffness is also increased, accounting for the increase in pulse wave velocity (PWV) toward the periphery. The mechanical behavior of peripheral vessels is greatly influenced by the behavior of the smooth muscle, particularly by its degree of activation.

## 2.2. Material Properties of the Arterial Wall: Elastin, Collagen, and Smooth Muscle Cells

Vascular stiffness is traditionally expressed in terms of Young's modulus of elasticity, which gives a simple description of the elasticity of the arterial wall. Young's modulus of elasticity $(E)$ is defined by the ratio of tensile stress $(\sigma_t)$ to tensile strain $(\varepsilon_t)$. When the relationship between stress and strain is a linear one (Fig. 2-5), then the material is said to be Hookean, or simply that it obeys Hooke's law of elasticity. This normally applies to a purely elastic material. It is only valid for application to a cylindrical blood vessel when the radial and longitudinal deformations are small, compared to the respective lumen diameter or length of the arterial segment.

For the following analysis of the physical aspect of an artery, we shall consider a segment of the artery represented by a uniform isotropic cylinder with radius, $r$, wall thickness, $h$, and segment length, $l$ (Fig. 2-6). Isotropy implies the uniform physical properties of the content of the arterial wall, which is actually anisotropic, consisting of the various components discussed above, but this assumption cannot be exactly true. Although a gross approximation, this assumption allows simple descriptions of the mechanical properties of the arterial wall to be obtained.

Young's modulus of elasticity, in terms of tensile stress and tensile strain is:

$$E = \sigma_t/\varepsilon_t \qquad (2\text{-}6)$$

Stress has the dimension of pressure, or force $(F)$, per unit area $(A)$,

$$\sigma_t = F/A = P \qquad (2\text{-}7)$$

where $P$ is pressure, in mmHg or dyn/cm$^2$. Thus, stress has the dimension of mmHg or dyn/cm$^2$ in cm,gm,s. The conversion of mmHg to dyn/cm$^2$ follows the formula that expresses the hydrostatic pressure above atmospheric pressure:

$$P = h\,\rho\,g \qquad (2\text{-}8)$$

where $h$ is the height of the mercury (Hg) column (Fig. 2-7), $\rho$ is the density of mercury, or 13.6 gm/cm$^3$, and $g$ is the gravitational acceleration. Hence 100 mmHg, or 10 cmHg, is equivalent to

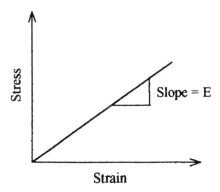

Fig. 2-5. Diagram illustrating the definition of the Young's modulus of elasticity with stress plotted on the ordinate and strain plotted on the abscissa . The stress–strain relation is a linear one, and the slope represents the elastic modulus, $E$.

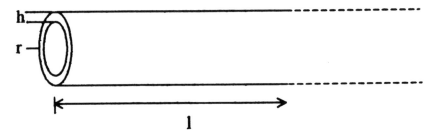

Fig. 2-6. Segment of an artery represented by a uniform isotropic cylinder, with lumen radius, $r$, arterial wall thickness, $h$, and segment length, $l$.

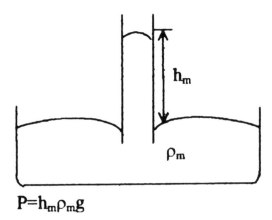

Fig. 2-7. Diagram defining hydrostatic pressure by a rising Hg column above the atmospheric pressure. Density of Hg is 13.6 g/cm³, the height $h$ in cm, and gravitational acceleration, $g$.

$$P = 100 \text{ mmHg} = 10 \times 13.6 \times 980 = 133,280 \text{ dyn/cm}^2 \quad (2\text{-}9)$$

or about $1.33 \times 10^5$ dyn/cm$^2$.

Strain in the longitudinal direction, or along the length of the blood vessel is expressed as the ratio of extension per unit length, or the ratio of the amount stretched longitudinally to the length of the original vessel segment,

$$\varepsilon_t = \Delta l / l \quad (2\text{-}10)$$

Strain in the radial direction, or perpendicular to the vessel segment length, is the fraction of distention of the vessel lumen radius or diameter. It is given by

$$\varepsilon_r = \Delta r / r \quad (2\text{-}11)$$

As an example, the radial strain, calculated from an ultrasonic dimension gage recording of the aortic diameter shown in Fig. 2-8, is

$$\varepsilon_r = 1.93/19.3 = 0.1 \quad (2\text{-}12)$$

In this case, the fractional change in diameter, or $\Delta D/D$, represents the radial strain.

For a blood vessel considered to be purely elastic, Hooke's law applies. To find the tension ($T$) exerted on the arterial wall caused by intraluminal blood pressure distention, Laplace's law is useful. Laplace's law was originally developed to describe the tension exerted on a curved membrane with a radius of curvature (Woods, 1892). In the case of blood vessel, there are two radii of curvature, one that is infinite in the longitudinal direction along the blood vessel axis, and the other in the radial direction. Thus, Laplace's law for an artery can be written as:

$$T = P\, r \quad (2\text{-}13)$$

This assumes the artery has a thin wall, or that the ratio of arterial wall thickness ($h$) to arterial lumen radius ($r$) is small, or h:r $\leq$ 1/10. Here $p$ is the intramural–extramural pressure difference, or the transmural pressure. When the arterial wall thickness is taken into account, the Lamé equation becomes relevant:

$$\sigma_t = pr/h \quad (2\text{-}14)$$

Arteries have been assumed to be incompressible. Although not exactly so, this is, in general, a good approximation. To assess the compressibility of a material, the Poisson ratio is defined. It is the ratio of radial strain to longitudinal strain. We obtain, from the above definitions, the Poisson ratio as:

$$\sigma = \frac{\varepsilon_r}{\varepsilon_t} = \frac{\Delta r / r}{\Delta l / l} \quad (2\text{-}15)$$

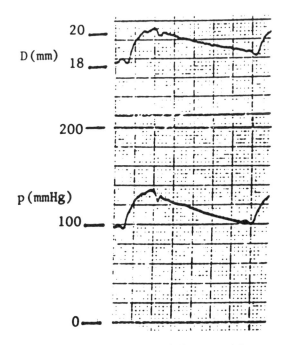

Fig. 2-8. Ultrasonic dimension gages recorded diameter of the aorta, together with aortic blood pressure. Calculation of radial strain can be obtained from the fractional change in diameter, $\Delta D/D$.

When radial strain is half that of longitudinal strain, or when $\sigma = 0.5$, the material is said to be incompressible. This means that, when a cylindrical material is stretched, its volume remains unchanged. Or, in the case of an artery, when it is stretched, its lumenal volume remains unchanged. Experimental measurements to obtain the Poisson ratio for arteries have shown $\sigma$ to be close to 0.5 (Carew et al., 1968). Arteries, therefore, can be considered to be close to being incompressible.

The above analysis assumes an isotropic arterial wall. The nonisotropy, or anisotropy, is seen in the various differences in the relative content and physical properties of the arterial wall. Collagen is the stiffest wall component, with an elastic modulus of $10^8$–$10^9$ dyn/cm$^2$ (Burton, 1954). This is about two orders of magnitude larger than those of elastin, $1$–$6 \times 10^6$ dyn/cm$^2$, and SM, $0.1$–$2.5 \times 10^6$ dyn/cm$^2$ (Bergel, 1961,1972; Hinke and Wilson, 1962).

Elastin is relatively extensible (Carton et al., 1962), but is not a purely Hookean material. Collagen, on the other hand, is relatively inextensible, because of its high stiffness. Much more is known about vascular smooth muscle (Somlyo and Somlyo, 1968). Smooth muscle can exert influence

## Small Artery

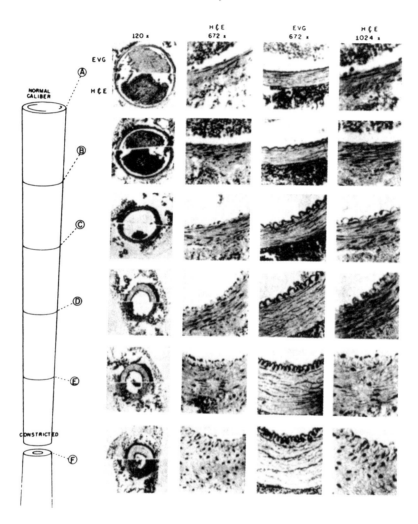

Fig. 2-9. Effects of vasoactivity on arterial lumen diameters. With vasoconstriction the lumen size decreases significantly (**A–F**), with corresponding increase in wall thickness. The relative changes in constituent components are also shown on the right panels. Adapted with permission from Rushmer (1972).

on large vessels, such as the aorta. Its activity in smaller arteries is greater, because of the increased wall thickness:radius ratio. With varied vasoactivity, arterial lumen can be modulated to regulate perfusion: Fig. 2-9 illustrates this. Considerable variations in the constituent wall components, collagen, elastin, and smooth muscle can be observed. Geometric change, such as the increased wall thickness to radius ratio is clearly visible.

Mechanical properties of arterial vessel walls can also be altered by neural mechanisms and by circulating catecholamines, such as norepinephrine (Aars, 1971). The composite of the arterial wall components operates in such a manner that, at low pressures, elastin dominates the composite behavior. At high pressures, collagen becomes more important. Elastic modulus is a nonlinear function of pressure. The pressure dependence of the mechanical properties of some arteries has been reported by several investigators (e.g., Cox, 1975; Li et al., 1990,1993; Li and Zhu, 1994; Drzewiecki et al., 1998). Figure 2-10 illustrates how arterial lumen diameter and compliance vary with changing transmural pressure. With increasing positive transmural pressure, arterial vessel diameter is distended, as expected, the corresponding compliance, however, declines. With negative transmural pressure, the arterial area compliance decreases as the artery is under collapse. The decrease in compliance with increasing transmural pressure follows a negative exponential function.

Along the arterial tree, longitudinally, we find that the number of elastic laminae decreases with increasing distance from the aorta, but the amount of smooth muscle increases and the wall thickness:radius ratio increases. The stiffness is thus increased, which accounts for the large increase in PWV (*see* Chapter 4). The mechanical properties are largely influenced by the behavior of the smooth muscle. Its elastic properties and activation are examined by, among others, Dobrin and Rovick (1969), Dobrin (1986), Herlihy and Murphy (1974), Apter et al. (1966), and Apter (1967).

A longitudinal section reveals a helical organization of the collagen fiber network, which contributes mostly to the anisotropic properties of the arterial wall. Its nonlinear property has been analyzed by Cheung and Hsiao (1972). The anisotropy of the arterial wall has been shown from rheological studies, and the stress–strain relationship was shown by Patel and Vaishnav (1972), Patel et al. (1969), and Oka (1981).

## 2.3. Viscoelastic Properties of Blood Vessels

Many investigators have examined static elastic properties of arteries (e.g., Bergel, 1961a; Peterson et al., 1960). It is found that the stress–strain, or length–tension relationship is nonlinear, and thus does not obey Hooke's law. Arterial elasticity increases with extension and the length–tension relation is curvilinear. Many experiments, however, were done in vitro, having the advantage of well-controlled experimental conditions, but having the disadvantage of extending the results to identify with corresponding in vivo parametric changes.

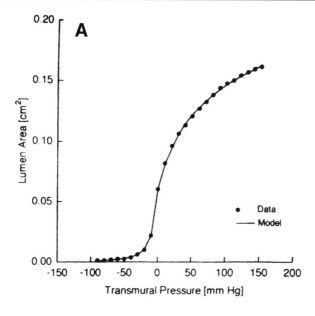

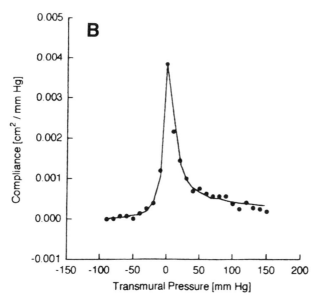

Fig. 2-10. Pressure dependence of mechanical properties of arteries is demonstrated in these figures. (**A**) Lumen diameter increases with transmural pressure, following an S-shape. (**B**) Area compliance plotted as a function of both positive and negative transmural pressures. Compliance decreases with increasing pressure, when the transmural pressure is positive, and when the vessel is collapsing with negative transmural pressure. Adapted with permission from Drzewiecki et al. (1997).

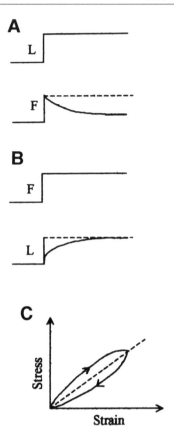

Fig. 2-11. Diagram illustrating the characteristics of a viscoelastic material such as the arterial wall: (**A**) stress relaxation: A step increase in length, *L*, or diameter, results in an increase in force or tension, which declines over time to a lower level, (**B**) creep phenomenon: With a step increment in applied force, the arterial length or diameter increases, but gradually; and (**C**) hysteresis; With increase in stress, strain increases, but when the stress is removed, the strain follows a different path, resulting in a hysteresis loop indicating energy loss. Provided by J. Xiao.

A purely elastic material differs from a viscoelastic material. The former depends only on strain (Eqs. 2-10 and 2-11); the latter depends on the rate of change of strain, or strain rate ($d\varepsilon/dt$) also. The artery as a viscoelastic material exhibits stress relaxation, creep, and hysteresis phenomena (Fig. 2-11).

If a strip of artery is subjected to a step change in length, it will result in an initial increase in stress, and then decays to a lower value. This is known as stress relaxation. There is a finite amount of time the vessel takes to relax. This is described by a time constant, which differs in different arteries. When an artery is subjected to a stepwise change in stress, its length will gradually increase to a constant value. This is the so-called "creep phenomenon." As with stress relaxation, the increase in length or diameter also takes a finite amount of time, and is also subscribed to a time constant. These properties allow arteries to respond to rapid transient changes in transmural blood pressures.

Hysteresis develops when the vessel is subjected to sinusoidal or cyclic changes. If the artery is purely elastic, there will be no phase shift between the applied pressure and the resulting change in diameter. The viscoelastic behavior of the artery leads to phase shifts in its pressure–diameter relation. A hysteresis loop is observed, reflecting viscous losses. In other words, energy is dissipated in stretching the artery, and allowing it to return to its control value. If the artery were purely elastic, there would be no energy loss and the artery would return to its control value along the exact path during stretching. Examples of experimentally measured pressure–diameter relations are shown in Fig. 2-12 for the pulmonary aorta. Because the pulmonary aorta is normally oval, there are two different diameters, namely, the major axis diameter and the minor axis diameter. When the major and minor axis diameters are plotted against pressure, the hysteresis loops are clearly seen. It is also clear that the pulmonary aorta is stiffer (less diameter distention with increasing pressure) along the major axis than along the minor axis. In small peripheral vessels, the viscous modulus is larger, and the phase shift becomes more pronounced. This can be seen, e.g., in the simultaneously measured pressure–diameter relation obtained for the femoral artery.

The static modulus of elasticity differs from the dynamic elastic value. Measurement of dynamic elasticity has gained considerable attention, chiefly because of its applicability to pulsatile conditions. The approach employs the measurement of pressure–diameter relations, and the subsequent calculations of the incremental elastic modulus ($E_{inc}$), which is complex ($E_c$):

$$E_{inc} = E_{dyn} + \eta\omega \qquad (2\text{-}16)$$

When the elastic modulus is complex, it implies frequency dependence. The in-phase component defines the dynamic elastic modulus,

$$E_{dyn} = |E_c| \cos\phi \qquad (2\text{-}17)$$

and the viscous modulus is defined by

$$\eta\omega = |E_c| \sin\phi \qquad (2\text{-}18)$$

where $\phi$ is the phase lag, generally between pressure ($p$) and diameter ($d$). When pressure leads diameter, or when the diameter distention delays after the arrival of the pressure pulse, $\phi$ is positive. When considering the artery as purely elastic, i.e., no viscosity damping is present, then the arterial lumen diameter changes instantaneously with the distending pres-

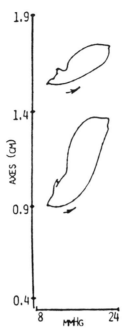

Fig. 2-12. Pressure-diameter relation of the main pulmonary artery showing hysteresis loops. Top tracing: major axis. Bottom tracing: minor axis. Adapted with permission from Li (1987).

sure pulse. In this case, $\phi$ is zero, and the viscous term $\eta\omega$ disappears. The phase angles are small in the aorta, and become larger in small, muscular arteries, such as the femoral.

A similar form of complex elastic modulus was given by Cox (1975), accounting for arterial wall thickness:

$$E(\omega) = \frac{4a^2 b}{b^2 - a^2} \frac{P(\omega)}{D(\omega)} \tag{2-19}$$

where a and b are inner and outer arterial diameters, respectively. $P(\omega)$ and $D(\omega)$ are frequency domain pressure and diameter, respectively.

Experimental results show that the viscous modulus is small, compared with the elastic modulus (Bergel, 1961; Gow and Taylor, 1968; Li et al., 1981; Li, 1987), on the order of 10%. The dynamic modulus has also been found to be essentially constant above 2 Hz (Fig. 2-13), an observation that, seen in Subheading 4.3., resembles the frequency-dependent behavior of PWV. This is, as mentioned before, because of its dependence on the properties of the arterial wall. Westerhof and Noordergraaf (1970) considered a complex Young's modulus to describe arterial wall viscoelasticity, and also utilized frequency-dependent parameters. They define the complex elastic modulus as the ratio of complex stress to complex strain:

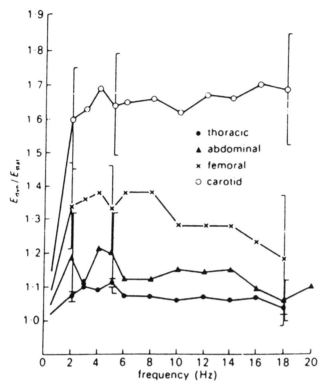

Fig. 2-13. Dynamic elastic modulus ($E_{dyn}$) plotted as a function of frequency for the thoracic aorta, abdominal aorta, and femoral and carotid arteries. Notice that the $E_{dyn}$ is essentially unchanged above 2 Hz.

$$E_c(\omega) = \frac{\sigma(\omega)}{\varepsilon(\omega)} \qquad (2\text{-}20)$$

$$E_c(\omega) = \frac{F(\omega)/A}{\Delta l(\omega)/l(\omega)} \qquad (2\text{-}21)$$

It is clear that, at $\omega = 0$, or when the elastic modulus is frequency-independent, this equation reduces to Eq. 2-6. $l(\omega)$ is the length, $F(\omega)$ is the sinusoidally applied force, and $\Delta l(\omega)$ is the change in length. In Laplace notation, they showed that, if a unit change in length in the form of a step function is applied to the Voigt model (Fig. 2-14), its force development (stress relaxation) is unbounded. When a unit change in force is applied to the Maxwell model (Fig. 2-14), its change in length (creep phenomenon) is unbounded. Thus, both models fail to represent adequately the physical properties of blood vessels. This indicates that a single time constant alone

VOIGT                    MAXWELL

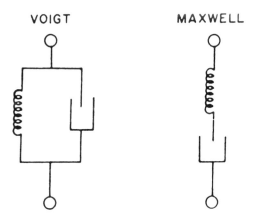

Fig. 2-14. Mechanical models of viscoelastic arteries. The spring–dashpot models are subjected to step changes in force, and step changes in length. In a Maxwell model, creep is unbounded; in a Voigt model, stress relaxation is unbounded.

is not sufficient to describe either the stress-relaxation or the creep phenomenon. Consequently, additional time constants have been suggested to be necessary. In order to sufficiently describe arterial viscoelasticity, Westerhof and Noordergraaf (1970) and Wessling et al. (1973) proposed a two-time-constants, five-element model of the arterial wall. With this model, they have shown that both stress relaxation and creep are bounded. Goedhard and Knoop (1973) extended this to a nine-element model. As more elements are incorporated, one obviously encounters difficulty in identifying their physiological counterparts.

## REFERENCES

Aars, H. Diameters and elasticity of the ascending aorta in normal and hypertensive rabbits. *Acta Physiol. Scand.* 83:133–138, 1971.

Apter, J. T. Correlation of visco-elastic properties of large arteries with microscopic structure. IV. Thermal responses of collagen, elastin, smooth muscle, and intact arteries. *Circ. Res.* 21: 901-918, 1967.

Apter, J. T., Rabinowitz, M., and Cummings, D. H. Correlation of viscoelastic properties of large arteries with microscopic structure. 1. Collagen, elastin, and smooth muscle determined chemically, histologically, and physiologically. *Circ. Res.* 19:104–121, 1966.

Bergel, D. H. Static elastic properties of the arterial wall. *J. Physiol.* 156:455–457, 1961.

Bergel, D. H. Dynamic elastic properties of the arterial wall. *J. Physiol.* 156:458–469, 1961.

Bergel, D. H. Properties of blood vessels. In: Fung, Y. C., ed., *Biomechanics,* Prentice-Hall, Englewood Cliffs, NJ, 1972.

Bloom, W. and Fawcett, D. W. A *Textbook of Histology.* Saunders, Philadelphia, 1975.

Burton, A. C. Relation of structure to function of the tissues of walls of blood vessels. *Physiol. Rev.* 34:619–642, 1954.

Carew, T. E., Vaishnav, R. N., and Patel, D. J. Compressibility of the arterial wall. *Circ. Res.* 22:61–68, 1968.

Carton, T. W., Dainanskas, J., and Clark, J. W. Elastic properties of single elastic fibers. *J. Appl. Physiol.* 17:5457–5551, 1962.

Cheung, J. B. and Hsiao, C. C. Nonlinear anisotropic viscoelastic stresses in blood vessels. *J. Biomech.* 5:607, 1972.

Cox, R. H. Pressure dependence of the mechanical properties of arteries in vivo. *Am. J. Physiol.* 229:1371–1375, 1975.

Dobrin, P. B. and Rovick, A. A. Influence of vascular smooth muscle on contractile mechanics and elasticity of arteries. *Am. J. Physiol.* 217:1644–1651, 1969.

Dobrin, P. B. Biaxial anisotropy of dog carotid artery: estimation of circumferential elastic modulus. *J. Biomech.* 19:351–358, 1986.

Drzewiecki, G., Field, S., Mubarak, I., and Li, J. K.-J. Effect of vascular growth pattern on lumen area and compliance using a novel pressure-area model for collapsible vessels. *Am. J. Physiol. (Heart & Circ. Physiol.)* 273:H2030–2043, 1997.

Goedhard, W. J. A. and Knoop, A. A. Model of the arterial wall. *J. Biomech.* 6:281–288, 1973.

Gow, B. S. and Taylor, M. G. Measurement of viscoelastic properties of arteries in the living dog. *Circ. Res.* 23:111–122, 1968.

Green, H. D. Circulatory system: physical principles. In: Glasser, O., ed., *Medical Physics,* vol. II, Year Book, Chicago, 1950.

Herlihy, J. T. and Murphy, R. A. Force-velocity and series elastic characteristics of smooth muscle from the hog carotid artery. *Circ. Res.* 34:461, 1974.

Hinke, J. A. M. and Wilson, M. L. Study of elastic properties of a 550 µ artery in vitro. *Am. J. Physiol.* 203:1153–1160, 1962.

Iberall, A. S. Anatomy and steady flow characteristics of the arterial system with an introduction to its pulsatile characteristics. *Math. Biosci.* 1:375–395, 1967.

Learoyd, B. M. and Taylor, M. G. Alterations with age in the viscoelastic properties of human arterial walls. *Circ. Res.* 18:278–192, 1966.

Li, J. K.-J. *Mammalian Hemodynamics: Wave Transmission Characteristics and Similarity Analysis.* Ph.D. dissertation, University of Pennsylvania, Philadelphia, 1978. University Microfilms, Ann Arbor, 1978.

Li, J. K.-J., Melbin, J., and Noordergraaf, A. Optimality of pulse transmission at vascular branching junctions. *Proc. 6th Int. Conf. Cardiovasc. Syst. Dynamics,* pp. 228–230, 1984.

Li, J. K.-J., Melbin, J., Riffle, R.A., and Noordergraaf, A. Pulse wave propagation. *Circ. Res.* 49:442–452, 1981.

Li, J. K.-J. *Arterial System Dynamics.* New York University Press, New York, 1987.

Li, J. K.-J. *Comparative Cardiovascular Dynamics of Mammals.* CRC Press, New York, 1996.

Li, J. K.-J., Cui, T., and Drzewiecki, G. Nonlinear model of the arterial system incorporating a pressure-dependent compliance. *IEEE Trans. Biomed. Eng.* BME-37:673–678, 1990.

Li, J. K.-J. Feedback effects in heart-arterial system interaction. *Adv. Exp. Med. Biol.,* 346:325–333, 1993.

Li, J. K-J. and Zhu, Y. Arterial compliance and its pressure-dependence in hypertension and vasodilation. *Angiology J. Vas. Dis.* 45:113–117, 1994.

Ling, S. C., Atabek, H. B., Fry, D. L., Patel, D. J., and Janicki, J. S. Application of heated film velocity and shear probes to hemodynamic studies. *Circ. Res.* 23:789–801, 1968.

McDonald, D. A. *Blood Flow in Arteries.* Arnold, London, 1974.

Oka, O. *Cardiovascular Hemorheology.* Cambridge University Press, New York, 1981.

Patel, D. J., Janicki, J. S., and Carew, T. E. Static anisotropic elastic properties of the aorta in living dogs. *Circ. Res.* 25:765–769, 1969.

Patel, D. J. and Vaishnav, R. N. Rheology of large blood vessels. In: Bergel, D. H, ed., *Cardiovascular Fluid Dynamics,* pp. 2–64, Academic, London, 1972.

Peterson, L. H., Jensen, R. E., and Parnell, J. Mechanical properties of arteries in vivo. *Circ. Res.* 8:622–639, 1960.

Rushmer, R. F. *Structure and Function of the Cardiovascular System.* Saunders, Philadelphia, 1972.

Somlyo, A. P. and Somlyo, A. V. Vascular smooth muscle, 1. Normal structure, pathology, biochemistry and biophysics. *Pharm. Rev.* 20:197–272, 1968.

Van der Werff, T. J. Significant parameters in arterial pressure and velocity development. *J. Biomech.* 7:437, 1974.

Wessling, K. H., Weber, H., and Dewit, B. Estimated five component viscoelastic model parameters for human arterial walls. *J. Biomech.* 6:13, 1973.

Westerhof, N., Bosman, F., DeVries, C. J., and Noordergraaf, A. Analog studies of the human systemic arterial tree. *J. Biomech.* 2:121–143, 1969.

Westerhof, N. and Noordergraaf, A. Arterial viscoelasticity: a generalized model. *J. Biomech.* 3:357–379, 1970.

Woods, R. H. A few applications of a physical theorem to membranes in the human body in a state of tension. *J. Anat. Physiol.* 26:362–370, 1892.

# 3 Theories and Models of Arterial Circulation

## 3.1. Simple Windkessel Model of the Arterial System

The simplicity of the windkessel model in interpreting pressure and flow behavior of the arterial tree has extended its use to much of last century. Modern development of theories in analyzing blood pressure and flow waveforms, and in explaining pulse transmission characteristics, have centered on the improvement of the original windkessel model. One of the shortcomings of the windkessel model is its lack of finite velocity of propagation. Finite pulse wave velocity (PVW) is discussed in the next subheading. We first look at the impact that the windkessel model has had on overall understanding of arterial circulation.

Lumped model of the arterial circulation was first described by Hales back in 1733. Although mostly qualitative, his model did emphasize the storage properties of large arteries and the dissipative nature of small peripheral resistance vessels. In this manner, the blood ejected by the heart during systole into the arterial system distends the large arteries (primarily the aorta). During diastole, the elastic recoil of these same arteries propels blood to perfuse the smaller peripheral resistance vessels. This thinking initiated the earlier conceptual understanding that the distensibility of large arteries is important in allowing the transformation of intermittent outflow of the heart to steady outflow throughout the peripheral vessels. In other words, the large compliance of the larger arteries protects the stiff peripheral vessels of organ vascular beds from the large swing of BP caused by pulsations. This latter view is still held by some until this day. The significance of arterial pulsations continues to be debated. The necessity of pulsatile perfusion, however, is well rooted, and demonstrated in both experimental and clinical studies.

Quantitative description of Hale's concept was not provided until Frank (1899,1926), whose interest originated in obtaining stroke volume, or the amount ejected by the ventricle per beat, from measured aortic pressure (AoP) pulse contour. Indeed, even decades later, methods to derive flow from pressure measurement or the so-termed pressure-derived flows (Fry and Greenfield, 1968; Li, 1983), continued to attract considerable interest

From: *Arterial Circulation: Physical Principles and Clinical Applications*
By: J. K-J. Li © Humana Press Inc., Totowa, NJ

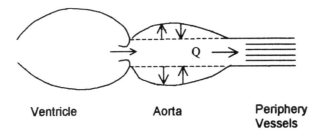

Ventricle                  Aorta                   Periphery
                                                  Vessels

Fig. 3-1. Diagrammatic representation of the LV and the arterial circulation, based on
the idea of the windkessel. The ventricle ejects into a compliant chamber representing
the aorta, blood flow is stored in systole (solid line), and, on elastic recoil in diastole
(dotted line), the stiff peripheral vessels are perfused.

until the advent of the popularity of electromagnetic blood flow and ultrasonic blood velocity measuring devices. Utilizing Frank's air-bellows
description of the arterial system, the ventricle ejects into a compliant
chamber representing the aorta, where blood flow is stored in systole, and,
on its elastic recoil in diastole, the stiff peripheral vessels are perfused.

In the windkessel analysis (e.g., Wetter and Kenner, 1968), the amount
of blood flow, $Q_s$, stored during each contraction, is the difference between
inflow, $Q_i$, to the large arteries and the outflow, $Q_o$, to the small peripheral
vessels (Fig. 3-1),

$$Q_s = Q_i - Q_o \qquad (3\text{-}1)$$

The amount of outflow is equivalent to the pressure drop from the arterial side $(P)$ to the venous side $(P_v)$ due to the peripheral resistance, $R_s$

$$Q_o = (P - P_v)/R_s \qquad (3\text{-}2)$$

At steady flow and assume that $P_v$ is small, we obtain a familiar expression for estimating the peripheral resistance, and with the total inflow, $Q$
$= Q_i$,

$$R_s = \overline{P}/\overline{Q} \qquad (3\text{-}3)$$

or mean arterial pressure to mean arterial flow. With pressure having the
unit of mmHg and flow in mL/s, the $R_s$ has the unit of mmHg/mL/s.

The storage property can be described by the use of arterial compliance,
which expresses the amount of change in blood volume $(dV)$ due to a
change in distending pressure $(dP)$ in the artery. In this case, we have

$$C = dV/dP \qquad (3\text{-}4)$$

Here $C$ represents the total compliance of the arterial system. With
volume measured in milliliters, then arterial compliance has the unit of

mL/mmHg. Peripheral resistance and arterial compliance have both remained the most popular parameters for clinical assessment of the properties of the arterial system.

The amount of blood flow stored, or $Q_s$, because of arterial compliance, is related to the rate of change in pressure distending the artery,

$$Q_s = C \, dP/dt \tag{3-5}$$

Substituting Eqs. 3-5 and 3-2 into 3-1, we obtain from

$$Q_i = Q_s + Q_o \tag{3-6}$$

an expression relating the arterial pressure to flow, incorporating the two windkessel parameters, $C$ and $R_s$:

$$Q(t) = C \, dP/dt + P/R_s \tag{3-7}$$

In other words, the total arterial inflow is the sum of the flow stored and the flow going into the periphery.

In diastole, when inflow is zero, as is the case when diastolic aortic flow equals zero, then

$$0 = C \, dP/dt + P/R_s \tag{3-8}$$

or

$$dP/P = -dt/R_s C \tag{3-9}$$

This equation states that the rate of diastolic aortic pressure drop is dependent on both the compliance of the arterial system and the peripheral resistance. Both of which also determine the flow. Integration of both sides of Eq. 3-9 gives us

$$\ln P = t/R_s C \tag{3-10}$$

or

$$P = P_o \, e^{-t/R_s C} \tag{3-11}$$

valid for the diastolic period, or $t = t_d$.

This last equation is seen to be equivalent to

$$P_d = P_{es} \, e^{-t_d/\tau} \tag{3-12}$$

or that the diastolic aortic pressure decay (Fig. 3-2) from end-systolic pressure ($P_{es}$) to end-diastolic pressure ($P_d$) follows a monoexponential manner, with a time constant of $\tau$. The time constant of pressure decay $\tau$, is determined by the product of resistance and compliance, i.e.,

$$\tau = R_s C \tag{3-13}$$

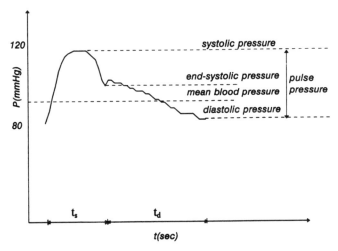

Fig. 3-2. Illustration of the measured aortic pressure pulse waveform. The systolic pressure, diastolic pressure, end-systolic pressure, and mean blood pressure are also shown. The approximate exponential decay of diastolic pressure through the diastolic period $(t_d)$ from the end of the systolic period $(t_s)$ is seen.

or, in terms of measured AoP,

$$\tau = \frac{t_d}{\ln \frac{P_{es}}{P_d}} \qquad (3\text{-}14)$$

This latter expression has been used extensively, and is a popular approach to estimate the total arterial compliance when peripheral resistance and aortic pressure pulse contour are known (*see also* Subheading 7.1.),

$$C = \frac{t_d}{R_s \ln \frac{P_{es}}{P_d}} \qquad (3\text{-}15)$$

Analysis, utilizing simple electric analog, has given the windkessel a two-element representation. Arterial compliance is represented by a capacitor, which has storage properties, in this case, electric charge. Peripheral resistance, with its viscous properties, is represented by a resistor that dissipates energy. The electrical analog of the windkessel model of the arterial system is shown in Fig. 3-3.

The two-element windkessel model was found to be insufficient to describe the vascular impedance to blood flow and to characterize the gross arterial tree properties. A modified windkessel model (Fig. 3-4), which has

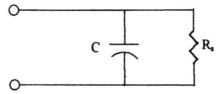

Fig. 3-3. The two-element resistance–capacitance electrical analog model of the windkessel. Compliance is represented by a capacitor, and the peripheral resistance by a resistor.

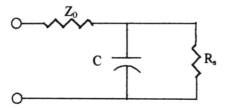

Fig. 3-4. An improved windkessel with three elements, with the addition of a pure resistance, $Z_o$, representing the characteristic impedance of the proximal aorta.

three-elements, was proposed by Westerhof et al. (1969). This lumped model of the systemic arterial tree has been widely used (Geipel and Li, 1990; Quick et al., 1995); it consists, in addition to arterial compliance and peripheral resistance of a characteristic impedance of the proximal aorta, termed $Z_o$, which is discussed in greater detail in Chapter 4. Its hydraulic equivalent is illustrated in Fig. 3-5.

### 3.2. Oscillatory Blood Flow in Arteries

It occurred to Euler (1775) that the pulse generated by the ventricle must propagate with a certain finite velocity. A mathematical formula, however, was developed initially by Young (1808). A similar expression was obtained by the Webers (e.g., 1850), who formulated three equations believed to be sufficient to characterize the propagation. The first of these equations is one that describes fluid motion,

$$\frac{\partial v_z}{\partial t} = \frac{1}{\rho} \frac{\partial p}{\partial z} \tag{3-16}$$

where $v_z$ is the blood velocity in the longitudinal $z$ direction or along the blood vessel from proximal to distal locations, $p$ is pressure, and $\rho$ is the density of blood, as before. The left side of the equation also represents the flow acceleration. This equation implies that blood flow acceleration is proportional to the pressure gradient. For this reason, this formula has been used to obtain blood flow from the measurement of pressure gradient.

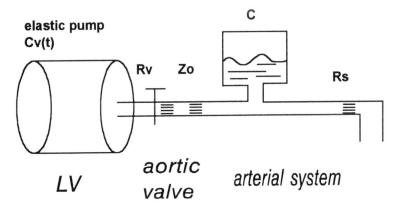

Fig. 3-5. The hydraulic equivalent of the three-element windkessel, popularly used to represent the arterial load to the heart. A bottle, allowing volume displacement subjected to pressure variations, represents arterial compliance. The peripheral resistance is represented by a needle valve whose partial opening and closing allows resistance to flow to be varied. The finite tube geometry and property represents the characteristic impedance of the aorta. Provided by Y. Zhu.

The second is the equation of continuity, to describe the incompressibility of the fluid:

$$\frac{\partial v_z}{\partial z} = \frac{1}{A}\frac{\partial A}{\partial t} = \frac{2}{r}\frac{\partial r}{\partial t} \tag{3-17}$$

or that blood flow velocity gradient is related to the rate of change in cross-sectional area of the blood vessel. In a cylindrical blood vessel, the cross-sectional area, $A$, is related to its inner lumen radius, $r$, as

$$A = \pi r^2 \tag{3-18}$$

Differentiate both sides with respect to time, we have

$$\frac{\partial A}{\partial t} = 2\pi r \frac{\partial r}{\partial t} \tag{3-19}$$

The third is the equation of state, to describe the elastic properties of the wall:

$$\frac{dr}{dp} = k \tag{3-20}$$

where $k$ is a constant. In other words, the pressure–radius relationship remains constant for the cardiac cycle.

From these, the Webers arrived at the wave equation, which gives the PWV:

$$c_o = \sqrt{\frac{r}{2k\rho}} \tag{3-21}$$

By defining Young's modulus of elasticity for the vessel, as in Chapter 2,

$$E = \frac{\sigma_t}{\varepsilon_r} \tag{3-22}$$

Resal (1876) independently found, using the Lamé equation, modified from Laplace's law accounting for wall thickness, $h$, for stress

$$\sigma_t = \frac{pr}{h} \tag{3-23}$$

and strain,

$$\varepsilon_r = \frac{dr}{r} \tag{3-24}$$

obtained a wave equation, giving the pulse wave velocity as

$$c_0 = \sqrt{\frac{Eh}{2r\rho}} \tag{3-25}$$

This formula for the purpose of the calculation of arterial PWV when the geometry and elasticity of the artery are known, is identical to the Moens-Korteweg formula. Moens (1878) obtained this formula through experimentation; Korteweg (1878) approached it from a theoretical perspective, by assuming a flat velocity profile, ignoring viscosity, fluid compressibility, and wall constraints.

The flat velocity profile implies that the blood flow velocity across the artery is uniform. In a parabolic velocity profile, the centerline velocity is the highest and the velocity declines in a parabolic fashion toward the vessel wall, so that, at the arterial wall, the velocity is the lowest (Fig. 3-6). In the arterial system, the velocity profile is relatively flat or blunt at the entrance to the arterial system, or at the ascending aorta, and becomes progressively parabolic when approaching smaller arteries.

Lamb (1898) later assumed an inviscid fluid contained within a thin-walled tube (wall thickness is small, compared to the lumen radius, i.e., $h << r$) subjected to small strains (ratio of radial distention to vessel radius, or $dr/r$, is small), and arrived at equations of motion for the wall in both the longitudinal and the radial directions. These equations were later incorporated by many investigators, notably Witzig (1914) and Womersley (1957).

Thus, arteries are subject to both longitudinal and radial tensions. According to Lamb, there are two modes of velocity of pulse propagation.

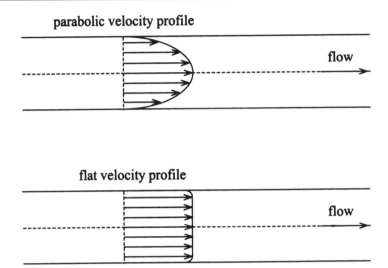

Fig. 3-6. Different velocity profiles. In a blunt or flat velocity profile (bottom tracing), the blood velocity across the vessel is uniform, and mostly found in large vessels, such as the proximal aorta. A parabolic velocity profile (top tracing) is when the centerline velocity is the highest with decreasing velocity toward the arterial wall occurring mosty in smaller arteries, such as the femoral. A skewed velocity profile occurs when the blood velocity is higher toward one wall than the opposite side.

One is identical to that given by the Moens-Korteweg formula, or Young's mode velocity of wave propagation, in which the wavelength of propagation is much greater, compared to the vessel radius ($\lambda \gg r$), and the blood and artery are both considered incompressible. The other is now known as the Lamb mode velocity for wave propagating longitudinally in the arterial wall:

$$c_0 = \sqrt{\frac{E}{\rho(1-\sigma^2)}} \qquad (3\text{-}26)$$

Wavelength is related to frequency and propagation velocity, as

$$\lambda = c/f \qquad (3\text{-}27)$$

For example, if the heart rate for a man is 60 beats/min (frequency is 1 Hz) and PWV in the human aorta is 500 cm/s, then the wavelength is

$$\lambda = 500/1 = 500 \text{ cm} \qquad (3\text{-}28)$$

which is considerably larger than the radius of the aorta (about 1.5 cm), or $\lambda \gg r$. With changes in heart rate and PWV, the ratio of $\lambda{:}r$ can vary considerably.

## 3.3. Linear Theories of Blood Flow in Arteries

Reviews of some of the linear theories are given by Noordergraaf (1969), Cox (1970), and Li (1987). Some of the modern theoretical development of blood flow in arteries can be traced back to Witzig's (1914) mathematical analysis who took into account the viscosity of the fluid, absent in wave equations obtained by previous proponents although this was done later by Morgan and Kiely (1954) who added viscous fluid to that presented by Lamb. Witzig's theoretical analysis became the basis of many modern pulse transmission theories. In general, linear theories regarding blood flow begin with the fundamental Navier-Stokes equations for a Newtonian and incompressible fluid (Attinger, 1964) in cylindrical coordinates, and assuming irrotational flow. Pulsatile pressure and flow relations, as well as complex velocity of wave propagation can be obtained (Noordergraaf, 1978; Li, 1987).

Differences in linearized theories are mostly in the description of arterial wall properties and arterial wall motion. More accurate descriptions of the blood–arterial wall interactions can be achieved by additions or improvements in the equations describing the wall and blood, or the so-called blood–wall interactions, which arise because of the fluid–tissue interface and the differences in mechanical behaviors. Indeed, modern clinical analysis has placed more emphasis on the blood–endothelial interface and on the blood flow and elastin-collagen interactions.

Of the many linear theories of blood flow in arteries, that of Womersley (1957) has become a popular one. A frequency-dependent parameter not originally defined by him, but later known as the Womersley's parameter, was introduced:

$$\alpha_w = r \sqrt{\frac{\omega \rho}{\eta}} \tag{3-29}$$

where $\omega = 2\pi f_h$, $f_h$ =heart rate; $\rho$ (1.06 g/cm$^3$) and $\eta$ (0.03 poise or 3 centipoise) are the density and viscosity of blood, respectively, and $r$ is the inner radius of the artery. This parameter also represents the ratio of the relative contribution of inertia component to viscous component of blood flow. In other words, it describes the ratio of the movement of blood mass to the retardation of flow or flow resistance caused by blood viscosity. $\alpha_\omega$ is also dependent on arterial lumen radius, thus, the smaller the vessel, the smaller the value of $\alpha_\omega$. Some examples of the magnitudes of $\alpha_\omega$ in arteries of man and dog are shown below:

| | | |
|---|---|---|
| Aorta (man): | $\alpha_\omega = 23$ | (3-30) |
| Aorta (dog): | $\alpha_\omega = 14$ | |
| Femoral artery (man): | $\alpha_\omega = 4$ | (3-31) |
| Femoral artery (dog): | $\alpha_\omega = 3$ | |

Thus, Womersley's parameter increases in magnitude with size of blood vessel and body weight (*see also* Subheading 7.4.).

In analyzing oscillatory blood flow in arteries, Womersley (1957) also utilized a linearized Navier-Stokes equation, and an equation of motion of a freely moving elastic tube with homogeneous and isotropic wall material. He also made assumptions that the pulse propagation wavelength is much greater than that of the arterial lumen radius, or $\lambda >> r$, and that the propagating pressure pulse takes the form of

$$p = A \, e^{\, j\omega \, (t-z/c)} \tag{3-32}$$

where $A$ is the magnitude of the pressure pulse and c is PWV.

An equation for the pulse wave velocity was derived, assuming arterial wall and blood densities are equal,

$$c = \sqrt{\frac{r\rho}{hE}} \, k_c \tag{3-33}$$

where $k_c$ is a function of the Bessel function

$$F_{10} = \frac{2J_1(\alpha j^{3/2})}{\alpha j^{3/2} \, J_0(\alpha j^{3/2})} \tag{3-34}$$

where $J_0$ and $J_1$, are zero and first order Bessel functions of the first kind. Solutions for $J_0$ and $J_1$ are tabulated by Womersley (1957) and van Brummelen (1961). Rewriting $F_{10}$ in its complex form in terms of real and imaginary parts, we have:

$$F_{10} = X + jY \tag{3-35}$$

Womersley obtained an expression for complex wave velocity:

$$c = \frac{1}{X-jY} \, \sqrt{\frac{Eh}{2r\rho}} \tag{3-36}$$

From this, the phase velocity is:

$$c_1 = \frac{c_0}{X} \qquad X = \frac{c_1}{c_0} \tag{3-37}$$

noting again that the Moens-Korteweg wave velocity is given by

$$c_0 = \sqrt{\frac{Eh}{2r\rho}} \tag{3-38}$$

The attenuation, expressed in terms of wavelength, is given by

$$\alpha_e = e^{-2\pi z Y/X\lambda} \tag{3-39}$$

Attenuation represents the degree of damping of the propagating pulse.

Womersley (1957) later imposed longitudinal constraint of the wall because of vessel tethering. In the case of infinite longitudinal constraint, $k_\infty$, wave velocity takes the form:

$$\frac{c_0}{c} = \sqrt{\frac{1-\sigma^2}{1-F_{10}}}$$

(3-40)

When considering the arterial wall as viscoelastic, the above equation is modified by taking into account the viscous property of the wall,

$$\frac{c_0}{c} = (X-jY)(1-j^1/_2\tan\phi)$$

(3-41)

It has been shown that the viscous component is relatively small in large arteries, such as the aorta. The viscous loss represented by the magnitude of $\tan\phi$ is less than 10%. Further discussion of attenuation and phase velocity can be found in Chapter 4.

Although inadequate, the Voigt model and the Maxwell model continue to be popular choices when taking into account of viscoelastic properties of the arterial wall. Viscoelasticity is discussed in Chapter 2. Womersley, as well as Morgan and Kiely (1954), Klip (1962), and Jager et al. (1965), employed the Voigt model to describe the arterial wall properties. Jager et al. (1965) also assumed a thick-walled model, when arterial wall thickness is a large fraction of the radius. A linearized Navier–Stokes equation and dynamic deformation of the wall were also incorporated, to arrive at a complex wave velocity:

$$c = \frac{Eh}{3\rho}\frac{2r+h}{(r+h)^2}(1-F_{10})$$

(3-42)

In general, pressure and flow are obtained as periodic solutions with spatial and temporal dependences as:

$$p(z,t) = M \cdot e^{j\omega(t-z/c)}$$

(3-43)

$$Q(z,t) = \frac{\pi r^2 M}{\rho c}(1-F_{10})e^{j\omega(t-z/c)}$$

(3-44)

Klip (1962) had earlier solved for phase velocity and damping for sinusoidal waves propagating in a thick-walled, homogeneous, isotropic viscoelastic wall containing viscous liquid. Cox (1968) later considered wave propagation in a freely moving, thick-walled viscoelastic tube containing Newtonian fluid; he summarized and compared linearized theories (Cox, 1970), as shown in Table 3-1.

Linear theories are based on certain assumptions, as discussed in the previous subheading, they are mathematically tractable, and allow solutions for pressure and flow to be expressed in closed forms.

Table 3-1
Comaprison of Linear Theories of Pulse Transmission

| General type and ref. | Incompressible fluid | Linear eqs. | Wall | | | | | | |
|---|---|---|---|---|---|---|---|---|---|
| | | | Thick | Rigid | Elastic | Visco-elastic | Isotropic | Incompressible | Inital stress |
| **Constrained** | | | | | | | | | |
| Witzig (1914) | + | + | 0 | 0 | + | 0 | + | 0 | 0 |
| Crandal (1927) | + | + | | + | 0 | 0 | | | 0 |
| Iberall (1950) | + | + | 0 | 0 | + | 0 | + | 0 | 0 |
| Womersley (1957) | + | + | 0 | 0 | + | 0 | + | 0 | 0 |
| Atabek (1968) | + | + | 0 | 0 | + | 0 | 0 | 0 | 0 |
| | | | | | | | | | |
| Maxwell and Anliker (1968) | 0 | + | 0 | 0 | 0 | 1 | + | 0 | + |
| Jones et al. (1968) | + | + | 0 | 0 | 0 | 1 | + | 0 | + |
| Jager et al. (1965) | + | + | + | 0 | 0 | 1 | + | + | 0 |
| Whirlow and Rouleau (1965) | + | + | + | 0 | 0 | 1 | + | 0 | 0 |
| Ling and Atabek (1972) | + | 0 | | 0 | + | 0 | + | | 0 |
| | | | | | | | | | |
| **Freely moving** | | | | | | | | | |
| Morgan and Kelly (1954) | + | + | 0 | 0 | 0 | 1 | + | 0 | |
| Womersley (1955) | + | + | 0 | 0 | + | 0 | + | 0 | 0 |
| Klip (1962) | 0 | + | 0 | 0 | 0 | 1 | + | 0 | 0 |
| Steerer et al. (1963) | + | * | 0 | 0 | + | | | | 0 |
| Atabek and Lew (1966) | + | + | 0 | 0 | + | 0 | + | 0 | + |
| Anlinker et al. (1968) | 0 | + | 0 | 0 | + | 0 | + | 0 | 0 |

| Model | | | | | | | | | |
|---|---|---|---|---|---|---|---|---|---|
| Barnard et al. (1966) | + | 0 | 0 | 0 | + | 0 | + | + | 0 |
| Chow and Apter (1968) | + | + | + | 0 | 0 | 2 | + | 0 | + |
| Klip et al. (1967) | + | + | + | 0 | 0 | 1 | + | 0 | 0 |
| Mirsky (1967) | + | + | * | 0 | + | 0 | 0 | 0 | 0 |
| Cox (1968) | + | + | + | 0 | 0 | 2 | + | + | 0 |
| Cos (1970) | + | + | + | 0 | 0 | 2 | + | 0 | 0 |

Adapted with permission from Cox (1970).

All models assume Newtonian fluid and laminar flow. All assume vicious fluid except Maxwell and Anliker (1968) and Anliker et al (1968).

Axisymmetric flow is assumed in all except Klip (1962) and Anliker et al. (1968).

+, indicates the assumption indicated at the head of the column; 0 means its absence; *, denotes a modified form of the assumption; 1, signifies a Voight model; 2, a standard linear solid model.

### 3.4. Analogy of Arterial Blood Flow to Transmission Line

The similarity of BF to the flow of electric current in transmission line cables have enabled the established voltage–current relation to be borrowed for the description of pressure–flow relation in arteries. The two- and three-element windkessel models discussed previously are, in effect, the lumped electrical analog models of the arterial circulation.

Arterial blood flow is analogous to a transmission line in that the solutions to pressure and flow, in the case of the blood vessel, and the solutions to voltage and current, in the case of the transmission line, are alike in their axial and time-dependent parts. For arteries, both longitudinal and transverse impedances are frequency-dependent.

A section of a linear electrical transmission line is shown in Fig. 3-7. The components are resistance, $R$, inductance, $L$, capacitance, $C$, and conductance or leakage resistance, $G$. The corresponding components for the circulation are resistance, inertance, arterial compliance, and resistance due to arterial wall viscosity, respectively. For this section, representative of an arterial segment, the constitutive equations are:

$$-\frac{\partial p}{\partial z} = (R' + j\omega L')Q \qquad (3\text{-}45)$$

$$-\frac{\partial Q}{\partial z} = (G' + j\omega C')p \qquad (3\text{-}46)$$

Equation 3-45 relates the pressure gradient, on the left hand side, to flow, on the right-hand side. Thus, knowing the resistance and inertia components, flow can be obtained from the knowledge of pressure gradient. In the catheterization laboratory, pressure gradient can be easily obtained through a heparinized saline-filled double-lumen catheter, or, alternatively, by a Millar-type catheter with dual sensors. The pressure gradient is estimated from the pressure difference

$$\Delta p = p_1 - p_2 \qquad (3\text{-}47)$$

over the sensor separation, $\Delta z$, or

$$\frac{dp}{dz} \approx \frac{\Delta p}{\Delta z} \qquad (3\text{-}48)$$

Similarly, Eq. 3-46 relates the flow gradient to pressure through arterial compliance and the viscous resistance elements. Frequently, these latter are used to provide a simple lumped representation of the viscoelastic properties of the artery.

For the ease of mathematical treatment, wave transmission through a uniform cylindrical tube of infinite length was studied by some investiga-

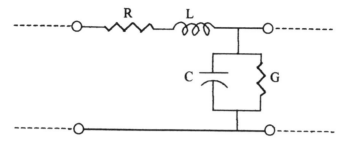

Fig. 3-7. Section of a linear transmission line showing the resistance, $R$, inductance, $L$, capacitance, $C$, and conductance or leakage resistance $G$.

tors. Arteries are of finite length. Consequently, it is more practical to consider segmental models. These latter circumvent the wave reflection effects (Subheading 4.4.). Womersley (1955) resolved this by relating pressure gradient to flow, and Jager (1965) utilized flow gradient to pressure. Both can be shown to be insensitive to wave reflections.

The impedance, or complex resistance to blood flow, along an artery is known as the longitudinal impedance, sometimes referred to as the fluid impedance, since only blood density and viscosity are involved, which is given by

$$Z'_l = \frac{-\partial p/\partial z}{Q} = R' + j\omega L' \qquad (3\text{-}49)$$

It is clear that resistance does not change with frequency, $\omega$, but that inductance does change with frequency. Thus, the longitudinal impedance can be obtained with the measurement of pressure gradient and flow, or the simultaneous measurements of two pressures separated by a small distance (e.g., 4–6 cm) and flow in an artery.

The transverse impedance, sometimes referred to as the arterial wall impedance, represents the impedance across the segment of an artery. The measurement of a flow gradient and a pressure suffice to determine the transverse impedance, i.e., the simultaneous measurements of two flow pressures separated by a small distance (e.g., 4–6 cm) and a pressure are required to determine transverse impedance. When the viscosity of the arterial wall is neglected, arterial compliance contributes solely to the transverse impedance, and we have

$$Z'_t = \frac{-p}{\partial Q/\partial z} = \frac{1}{j\omega C'} \qquad (3\text{-}50)$$

Thus, compliance of an arterial segment can be determined in this fashion, i.e., from the ratio of pressure to flow gradient. Of course, there are other means for determining arterial compliance, such as from the pressure–volume (P-V) relation.

Since both longitudinal and transverse impedances are components of the segment, they also bear the characteristics of the arterial segment. For this reason, a characteristic impedance, $Z_o$, can be defined in terms of them, i.e.:

$$Z_o = \sqrt{Z_l \cdot Z_t} \qquad (3\text{-}51)$$

$Z_o$, the characteristic impedance, by this definition, is therefore independent of distal or proximal pressure and flow changes, and is solely dependent on local fluid and mechanical properties. The pressure and flow pulse propagation through this segment is also dependent on these local longitudinal and transverse impedances. The local propagation constant of the arterial segment is

$$\gamma = \sqrt{Z_l/Z_t} \qquad (3\text{-}52)$$

Therefore, knowing the characteristic impedance and the propagation constant, the pulse propagation through the arterial segment can be defined. Propagations constant and chrarcteristic impedance require the simultaneous measurements of two pressures and two flows, which is not an easy experimental task (Li et al., 1981). These equations characterize pulse transmission through an arterial segment, represented by Fig. 3-8.

A wave equation that describes the pressure pulse propagation is given by

$$\frac{\partial^2 p}{\partial z^2} = \gamma^2 p \qquad (3\text{-}53)$$

where $\gamma$ is the propagation constant (Chapter 4), and the solution for pressure is:

$$p(z) = p_f e^{-\gamma z} + p_r e^{\gamma z} \qquad (3\text{-}54)$$

where $p_f$ is the forward or antegrade traveling pressure component away from the heart, and, $p_r$ is the reflected or retrograde traveling pressure component. Wave reflections are dealt with in greater detail in Chapter 4.

A corresponding equation for flow is:

$$Q(z) = \frac{1}{Z_o} (p_f e^{-\gamma z} - p_r e^{\gamma z}) \qquad (3\text{-}55)$$

Thus, flow through an arterial segment is determined by the geometric and mechanical properties of the segment and the forward and reflected pressure waves. It can be seen from the plus (+) and minus (−) signs that wave reflection has opposite effects on pressure and flow. Increased reflection increases pressure, but decreases flow. In the absence of wave

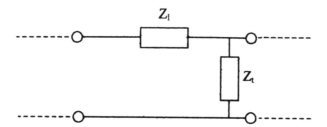

Fig. 3-8. Arterial segment represented by the longitudinal impedance, $Z_l$, and the transverse impedance, $Z_t$.

reflection ($p_r = 0$), pressure and flow are related by the characteristic impedance, $Z_o$, only. The mechanical properties of the segment embedded in the characteristic impedance and propagation constant, however, are independent of wave reflections.

## 3.5. Distributed and Reduced Arterial Tree Models

In the windkessel model, the arterial tree was considered to consist of the proximal aorta as a compliant vessel, with storage properties and peripheral vessels as stiff tubes that drain blood during the diastole. This results in a two-element electric analog model, as shown in Fig. 3-3. Westerhof et al. (1969) improvised on this to provide a reduced model that better explained the input impedance (Chapter 4) of the arterial tree; this modified windkessel model is shown in Fig. 3-4. The characteristic impedance of the aorta is represented by $Zo$, a frequency-independent resistance; compliance is represented by $C$ and $R_s$, represents the total peripheral resistance. The windkessel model is a valid representation of the input impedance only at low frequencies (*see* Chapter 4).

An electrical analog model of the human systemic arterial tree was given by Westerhof et al. (1969), as shown in Fig. 3-9. This model is based on linear transmission line theories, but incorporates viscoelastic elements. Each box shown represents an arterial segment. Pressure and flow waveforms can be obtained at a specified arterial site, in terms of voltage and current. Detailed description of the model and its utilization can be found in the text by Noordergraaf (1978), who also provided a reduced model of the systemic arterial tree (Fig. 3-10). Pollack et al. (1968) gave an analog model of the pulmonary arterial tree, a reduced model of which was given by Gopalakrishnan (1977), and was described by Li (1987), as in Fig. 3-11. The distributed models retain features that would otherwise be lost in the lumping process.

There are several other models of interest. O'Rourke (1967) and Avolio et al. (1976) proposed a T-shaped model representing upper and lower

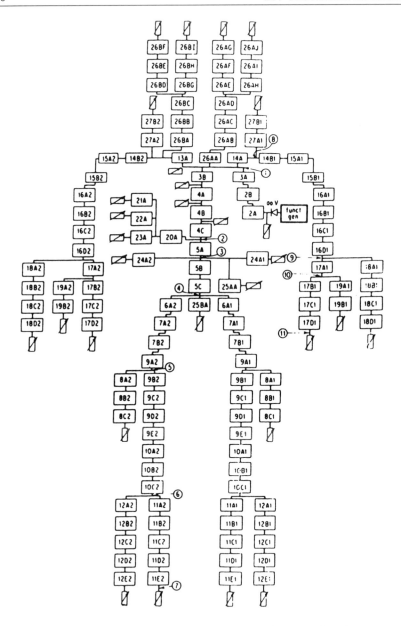

Fig. 3-9. Analog model of the human systemic arterial tree. A function generator generates the pressure pulse (voltage), which propagates through each segment, which are terminated by a lumped windkessel. The model was modified from elastic arteries to include viscoelastic properties of arteries (compliance–resistance or capacitor–resistor combination). This model allows pressure-flow relations, hence impedance, to be obtained at each arterial segment. Adapted with permission from Westerhof et al. (1969).

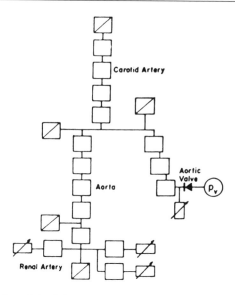

Fig. 3-10. Reduced model of the systemic arterial tree. This model includes pulse wave transmission in selected parts of the system. $P_v$ = ventricular pressure.

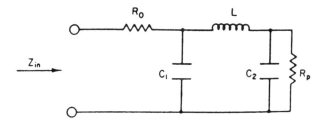

Fig. 3-11. Reduced model for the input impedance of the pulmonary arterial tree.

vascular sites (Fig. 3-12). These authors used the model to explain pressure and flow waveforms in relation to the anatomical design of the mammalian arterial system in the upper and lower parts of the body. The progressive morphological changes in pressure waveforms are also shown. This model was later modified to infer wave reflections at the aortic root by Burratini and Campbell (1989). The time-domain formulation of the assymmetric T-tube model was described by Campbell et al. (1990), and a single homogeneous tube model was provided by McDonald (1960). The single uniform tube model has been popular, mostly because of its simplicity. Two-tube models were proposed by Caro and McDonald (1961) and Kenner and Wetterer 1962); a three-tube model was later reported by Bauer et al. (1973). A nonuniform elastic tube model was given by Taylor (1966), to

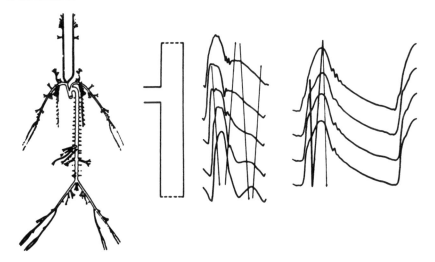

Fig. 3-12. T-tube model representing the upper and lower body arterial circulations. Adapted with permission from O'Rourke and Yaginuma (1984).

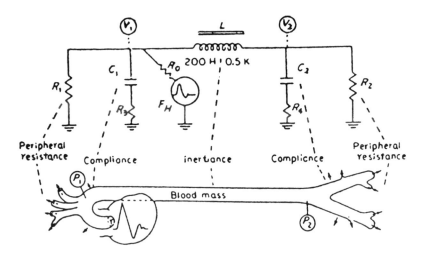

Fig. 3-13. Lumped model of the systemic arterial tree. Compliance and resistance at corresponding anatomic sites are shown. The inertance, $L$, represents blood mass associated with flow.

include spatial changes in arterial elasticity and geometry. Spencer et al. (1961) also provided a lumped model for the arterial tree, as shown in Fig. 3-13.

Rideout and Dick (1967) gave an analog computer model. Finkelstein et al. (1985) later proposed a similar model, in which arterial compliance is split into large-vessel and small-vessel compliances.

Digital computer models, however, have become popular in recent years, chiefly for their ease in handling parametric adjustment and simulation. For example, Stegiopoulos et al. (1992) developed a computer model and applied it to the simulation of the pressure and flow characteristics in aortic and arterial stenoses.

## 3.6. Nonlinear Aspects and Pressure-Dependent Arterial Compliance

Although the Navier-Stokes equation in its complete form has recently been solved in closed form (Melbin and Noordergraaf, 1982), there are other kinds of nonlinearities. Thus, depending on the particular problem or application at hand, assumptions included to eliminate certain other nonlinearities may still be valid for providing a satisfactory solution. This is particularly true regarding to the use of Fourier analysis in studying pressure and flow waveforms and the derived input impedance (Subheading 4.2.), but we shall examine some of the nonlinearities that have entered into pulse transmission analysis.

In Chapter 2, we see that arterial walls exhibit anisotropic characteristics of mechanical nonuniformity. Arteries do not obey Hooke's law, except for small strains. Shear stress is a function of radial strain, and increases with increasing radius, as a result of pulsating pressure and differential elasticities of smooth muscle, elastin, and collagen. At higher pressures, arterial elasticity becomes a strong function of pressure (Fig. 3-14), i.e., $E = E(P)$. Thus, blood vessel is less extensible at higher pressures. It has been suggested that elastin dominates arterial wall behavior at low to normal levels of BP, but, at high BPs, collagen dominates the overall behavior. Smooth muscle activation can significantly alter the arterial wall contraction, as demonstrated in Fig. 3-15. Contraction is stronger in the presence of norepinephrine. When smooth muscle tone is abolished, e.g., with potassium cyanide, collagen properties become dominant, and the overall elasticity is greater.

This is also seen from measured wave velocity (Nichols and McDonald, 1972; Van den Bos et al., 1976). Pulse wave velocity increases with increasing mean blood pressure (Fig. 3-16); thus, arterial compliance is a function of pressure, i.e., $C = C(P)$, assumed constant by linear theories.

The general definition of arterial compliance is the ratio of an incremental change in volume resulting from an incremental change in distending pressure, i.e.,

$$C = dV/dP \tag{3-56}$$

This is defined by the inverse of the slope of the P-V curve, with pressure plotted on the ordinate and volume on the abscissa (Fig. 3-17). Thus, compliance is the inverse of elastance. The P-V curves of arteries have

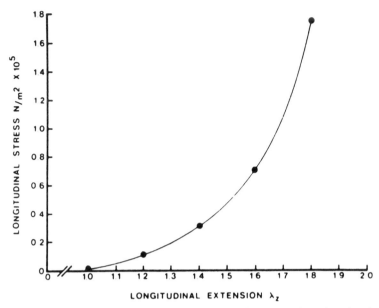

Fig. 3-14. Longitudinal stress plotted against longitudinal extension, showing that the stress-strain relation is curvilinear, and the proportional extension is less at higher stress. Adapted with permission from Dobrin (1986).

been found to be curvilinear. The slope changes along the P-V curve, steeper at higher pressures, signifying increased arterial stiffness or decreased compliance and distensibility. In other words, arteries stiffen when pressurized. This physiological phenomenon has been observed in many experiments. This increased stiffness has been suggested to be related to the structure of the arterial wall and implies that the compliance–pressure relation is not a constant one. Declining arterial compliance with increasing pressure has been observed in the central aorta and in individual arteries. The inverse exponential relations between compliance and pressure for the whole arterial system and for the femoral artery are shown in Figs. 3-18 and 3-19.

The pressure dependence of arterial compliance has been known for some time (e.g., Li et al., 1986,1990). It is still, however, considered a constant value in many model-based studies (e.g., Simon et al., 1979; Laskey et al., 1990; Stergiopoulos et al., 1994). The most popularly used model of the arterial system, the windkessel (Frank, 1899), for instance, is based on a linear P-V relation incorporating a constant elastic modulus. This assumes that the compliance of the arterial system remains constant throughout the cardiac cycle, in which compliances in systole and in diastole are assumed to be the same, despite varying pressure amplitudes

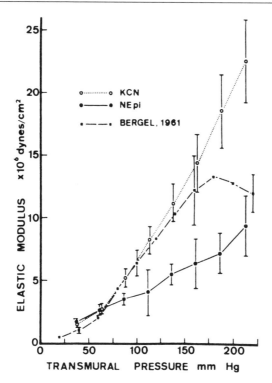

Fig. 3-15. Elastic modulus plotted as a function of transmural blood pressure. Increase in elastic modulus is more rapid at higher BP than at lower BP. The intramural stress–circumferential length diagrams for the carotid artery (dog) shows curvilinear increasing strain with increasing stress. The strong state of contraction caused by norepinephrine (Nepi), and when the smooth muscle tone is abolished by potassium cyanide (KCN), are shown. The difference between the two curves is the force developed by the active muscle. Adapted with permission from Dobrin and Rovick (1969).

(pulse pressure). We have shown that pulse pressure is a significant determinant of arterial compliance, even within a single cardiac cycle (Li and Zhu, 1994). This implies the inadequacy of the constant compliance models to accurately describe the arterial compliance behavior. Aside from the P-V curves, studies on pressure–strain elastic modulus ($Ep$) in the aorta have also shown the increase in $Ep$ with increasing pressure (Peterson et al., 1960; Li et al., 1986; Li, 1987),

$$Ep = (\Delta P/\Delta D) \cdot D \qquad (3\text{-}57)$$

where $\Delta p$ is the pulsatile arterial distending pressure and $\Delta D$ the corresponding pulsatile change in vessel diameter, and $D$ is the mean diameter. This formula assumes the blood vessel is thin-walled. Using a thick-walled model of arteries, taking into account arterial wall thickness, Cox (1975)

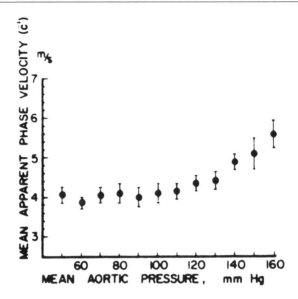

Fig. 3-16. Illustration of pressure dependence of PWV. The mean apparent phase velocity plotted as a function of mean blood pressure. Adapted with permission from Nichols and McDonald (1972).

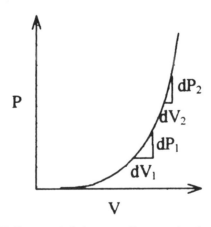

Fig. 3-17. Arterial P-V diagram, defining compliance as the slope of the relation ($C = dV/dP$). It is clear that the slope changes with increasing pressure ($dV_1/dP_1$ vs $dV_2/dP_2$) and that at higher pressures, the volume change is smaller.

also found the pressure dependence to be true. In addition, it was found that the degree of pressure dependence differs in different arteries. Simultaneous measurement of pulsatile pressure and diameter in the aorta demonstrated that, at elevated pressures, the pressure-strain $E_p$ is considerably greater.

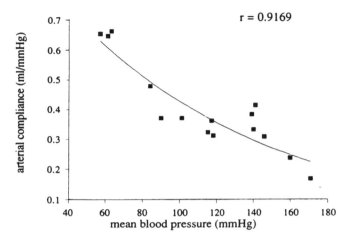

Fig. 3-18. Compliance plotted against mean arterial blood pressure reflecting the P-V relation. The relationship is nonlinear, implying that, at higher distending pressures, the intraluminal volume change is smaller, resulting in a lower compliance. The decrease in arterial compliance with increasing BP follows a negative exponential function.

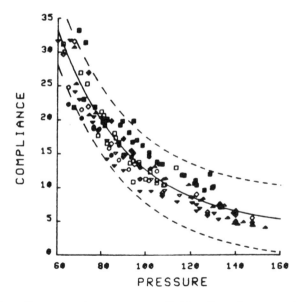

Fig. 3-19. Compliance as an inverse exponential function of pressure obtained in the femoral artery. Adapted with permission from Megerman et al. (1986).

The study of the pressure-dependent behavior of arterial compliance or vascular stiffness is important, because of its relevance to many cardiovascular diseases. Some of these are results of alterations in the mechanical properties of the vessel wall and vascular states. In hypertension, for instance, the increased pressure is always associated with a reduced arterial compliance (e.g., Randall et al., 1984; Li et al., 1986; Meister et al., 1992; Simon et al., 1992; Trazzi et al., 1993; Ting et al., 1993; Li and Zhu, 1994; for more details *see* Chapter 7). A decreased compliance can occur as a consequence of an elevated arterial pressure and that increased BP can result from a decreased compliance as a result of alterations in vessel wall properties.

A recently developed nonlinear model of the arterial system incorporating a pressure-dependent compliance element ($C(P)$) is shown in Fig. 3-20 (Li et al., 1990; Li, 1993; Li et al., 1994). The model consists of the characteristic impedance of the proximal aorta ($Z_o$), the peripheral resistance ($R_s$), and $C(P)$. The compliance is exponentially related to pressure, and is expressed as

$$C(P) = a \cdot e^{bP(t)} \tag{3-58}$$

where a and b are constants. The exponent b is normally negative. Thus, an inverse relationship is established between arterial compliance and BP; with increasing BP arterial compliance decreases.

Figure 3-20 shows that the flow through the compliance branch of the nonlinear model is given by

$$Qc(t) = Q(t) - P(t)/Rs \tag{3-59}$$

where $P(t)$ and $Q(t)$ are the pressure and flow through the compliance branch, respectively. This flow can also be expressed as

$$Qc(t) = C(P) \cdot dP(t)/dt \tag{3-60}$$

Equate these two equations (3-59 and 3-60), resulting in

$$dP/dt = Q(t) - P(t)/R_s/C(P) \tag{3-61}$$

This equation defines the dynamic relationship between pressure and flow for a nonlinear compliance element. Numerical methods can be employed to solve this equation.

Using difference representations, we have

$$\Delta t = t_{i+1} - t_i = dt \tag{3-62}$$

where $\Delta t$ is the sampling interval, taken as 10 ms. The nonlinear model is then reduced to the following expression:

$$P(t_{i+1}) = P(t_i) + \Delta t \times [Q(t_i) - P(t_i)/R_s]/C(P) \tag{3-63}$$

With the measured aortic flow as the input, a numerical procedure can be programmed to solve $P(t_i)$, $C(P)$, and the AoP

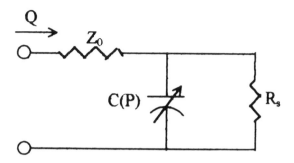

Fig. 3-20. Nonlinear arterial system model, incorporating a pressure-dependent compliance. $Z_o$ is characteristic impedance of the ascending aorta, $R_s$ is total peripheral resistance, $C(P)$ is the pressure-dependent compliance, represented by a variable capacitor. $Q$ is aortic flow.

$$P_a(t_i) = Q(t_i) \cdot Z_o + P(t_i) \qquad (3\text{-}64)$$

Aortic characteristic impedance was determined in the time domain from the instantaneous ratio of the upstroke of aortic pressure and flow above their respective end-diastolic levels during the early part of systole (Li, 1986):

$$Zo = \frac{P_a(t_i) - P_d}{Q_a(t_i)} \qquad (3\text{-}65)$$

where $P_d$ is the diastolic aortic pressure. The above equation was plotted for the first 60 ms of pressure and flow data, sampled at 10 ms intervals, and the average value of this ratio was obtained as $Z_o$. This time-domian approach was later applied to estimate aortic characteristic impedance in humans (Lucas et al., 1988). With strong vasodilation, such as intravenous infusion of nitroprusside, the effect of wave reflection can be mostly abolished. In this case, the relation of ascending aortic pressure to flow is linear, and its slope is a very good estimate of characteristic impedance (*see* Chapter 4).

The peripheral resistance was calculated from the ratio of mean pressure to mean flow,

$$Rs = \overline{P}/\overline{Q} \qquad (3\text{-}66)$$

In order to solve Eq. 3-63, several steps were taken. Aortic flow obtained from animal experimental data was used as input. Initial values of a and b were first estimated, based on curve-fitting of windkessel model compliance vs pressure data obtained for a number of beats. The initial value of $P(t)$ was chosen as $P_d$. This set of initial values were adjusted until the least-squares error, $E$, between measured and predicted AoP is minimized to meet the desired error within physiological limits,

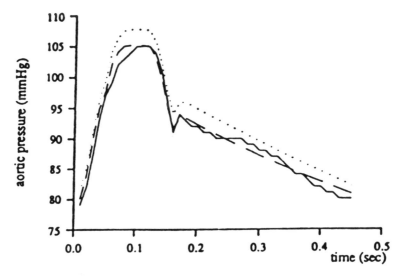

Fig. 3-21. Nonlinear pressure-dependent, compliance model-predicted AoP (dashed line), and the three-element, linear windkessel-model-predicted pressure (dotted line) and the measured pressure (solid line) are shown. The nonlinear model can more accurately predict the aortic pressure waveform. Provided by Y. Zhu.

$$E = \sum_{i=1}^{N} [P_a\text{calculated}(t_i) - P_a\text{measured}(t_i)]^2 \qquad (3\text{-}67)$$

where $N$ is the total number of sampled points within one complete cardiac cycle.

This nonlinear model predicted AoP accurately, as shown in Fig. 3-21. The linear three-element model predicted the measured AoP with less accuracy, although the gross features are evident. The model-based arterial compliance, plotted as a function of pressure for a complete cardiac cycle with a normal BP level, is shown in Fig. 3-22. It is clear from this figure that compliance is relatively independent of both pressure and flow in the early systole, and maintains a value close to its maximum during this period. This facilitates early rapid ventricular ejection. During mid-systole, arterial compliance begins to decline: This corresponds to increased AoP and reduced ejection after peak ventricular outflow. In the late systolic phase, arterial compliance declines rapidly, with a concurrent rapid decline of aortic flow, despite a falling AoP. The compliance value is much higher at early systole than at late systole. Arterial system compliance reaches its minimum at the end of the ejection. For the diastolic period, when aortic flow is zero, compliance follows an exponential relation, as given by Eq. 3-58. Its value increases throughout the diastole toward maximum, readying for the following ventricular ejection.

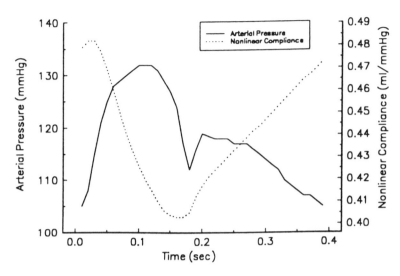

Fig. 3-22. Nonlinear pressure-dependent characteristics of arterial compliance as a function of time plotted for a complete cardiac cycle. Arterial compliance increases initially at the beginning of ejection and declines with increasing pressure. It reaches a minimum at about end-systole, and increases steadily, thence toward the end of diastole.

In describing fluid motions with a linearized Navier-Stokes equation, nonlinear terms are assumed to be small, and are consequently neglected. Ling et al. (1972,1973) computed flows from an accurately measured pressure gradient (with a claimed resolution of 0.001 mmHg) and found that linear theory overestimated the steady-flow term by several-fold; the pulsatile flow waveforms conformed well with electromagnetically measured flow. In linear transmission expressions, the steady-flow component is separate from oscillatory (harmonic) components in the Fourier series expansion, and hence does not contribute to pulse propagation.

Li et al. (1981) measured the propagation constant in arteries, and found that the measured attenuation coefficients and phase velocities differed greatly from those predicted by linear theories. To explain the observed discrepancies, they evaluated and compared the nonlinear and linear theories for the femoral artery. For the nonlinear theory, the complete solution of the Navier-Stokes equation, the geometric taper, and pressure-dependent wall compliance were incorporated. The linear model was taken as that of the three-element windkessel. Input parameters for the two models are shown in Table 3-2. Results of the contribution of individual Navier-Stokes terms to the pressure change, over 10 cm, are shown in Table 3-3. It can be seen that convective acceleration terms contributed little. Wall compliance largely overcome the effect of small geometric taper, which is

Table 3-2
Parameter Values for Nonlinear Femoral Model and its Linearized Version

| System parameter | Femoral model | Linear model |
|---|---|---|
| Fluid density ($\rho$, g/mL) | 1.055 | 1.055 |
| Fluid viscosity ($\mu$, poise) | 0.032 | 0.032 |
| Cycle period (t, s) | 0.576 | 0.576 |
| Vessel length (z, cm) | 10 | 10 |
| Taper constant (k) | 0.02 | 0 |
| Inner radius ($r_i$, cm) | 0.23 exp($-kz$) | 0.22 |
| Compliance ($dr_i/dp$, cm/mmHg) | 0.0019 exp($-kz$) (p)$^{-1/2}$ | $1.5 \times 10^{-4}$ |

Table 3-3
Contribution of Individual Navier-Stokes Terms to Pressure Change Over 10 cm

| Navier-Stokes term | Femoral model (mmHg) (% total) | Linear model (mmHg) (% total) |
|---|---|---|
| Viscous | | |
| $\mu\partial^2 v_z/\partial r^2$ | −0.553 (67.3) | −0.443 (71.9) |
| $\mu (1/r)\partial v_z/\partial r$ | −0.169 (20.6) | −0.136 (22.1) |
| $\mu\partial^2 v_z/\partial z^2$ | 0 (0.06) | 0 |
| Inertial | | |
| $\rho\partial v_z/\partial t$ | 0.033 (4) | −0.037 (6.1) |
| $\rho v_z\partial v_z/\partial z$ | −0.046 (5.6) | 0 |
| $\rho v_r\partial v_z/\partial r$ | −0.02 (2.4) | 0 |

more significant in large vessels, such as the aorta. Figure 3-23 shows pressures, flows, and their harmonic contents evaluated by the linear and nonlinear theories. The attenuation coefficients measured by different investigators and computed by linear and nonlinear theories are discussed in the following chapter. When linear equations are utilized, attenuation is attributed to viscous losses only. Thus, when experimental measurements are used with linear models, the viscous losses are artificially increased by the interpretation.

There are other forms of nonlinearities. For instance, turbulence and skewed velocity profiles associated with arterial blood flow rather than laminar flow with parabolic profile occur in some arterial sites. Although varied nonlinearities have been incorporated in some nonlinear theories, in general vascular branching has not been included. Its effect is significant in pulse transmission. This is discussed in Chapters 4 and 6.

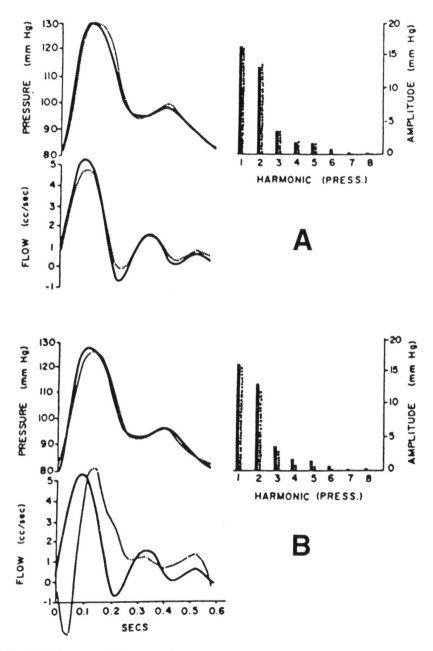

Fig. 3-23. Pressure and flow waveforms and harmonic contents computed from linear and nonlinear theories for the femoral artery. Nonlinear theories accounted for compliance as a function of pressure, and included nonlinear terms in the Navier-Stokes equations.

# REFERENCES

Attinger, E. O. *Pulsatile Blood Flow*. McGraw-Hill, New York, 1964.

Avolio, A. P., O'Rourke, M. F., Mang, K., Bason, P. T., and Gow, B. S. Comparative study of pulsatile arterial hemodynamics in rabbits and guinea pigs. *Am. J. Physiol.* 230:868–875, 1976.

Barnard, A. C. L., Hunt, W. A., Timlake, W. P., and Varley, E. Theory of fluid flow in compliant tubes. *Biophys. J.* 6:717–724, 1966.

Bauer, R. D., Pasch, T., and Wetterer, E. Theoretical studies on the human arterial pressure and flow pulse by means of a non-uniform tube model. *J. Biomech.* 6:289, 1973.

Burattini R. and Campbell, K. B. Modified assymemtric T-tube model to infer arterial wave reflection at the aortic root. *IEEE Trans. Biomed. Eng.* 36:805–814, 1989.

Campbell, K. B., Burattini, R., Bell, D. L., et al. Time domain formulation of assymmetric T-tube model of arterial system. *Am. J. Physiol.* 258:H1761–1774, 1990.

Caro, C. G. and McDonald, D. A. Relation of pulsatile pressure and flow in the pulmonary vascular bed. *J. Physiol.* 157:426-453, 1961.

Chang, C. C. and Atabek, H. B. Inlet length for oscillatory flow and its effects on the determination of the rate of flow in arteries. *Phys. Med. Biol.* 6:303–317, 1961.

Chow, J. C. and Apter, J. T. Wave propagation in a viscous incompressible fluid contained in a flexible viscoelastic tube. *J. Acoust. Soc. Am.* 44:437–443, 1968.

Cox, R. H. Comparison of linearized wave propagation models for arterial blood flow analysis. *J. Biomech.* 2:251-265, 1970.

Cox, R. H. Pressure dependence of the mechanical properties of arteries in vivo. *Am. J. Physiol.* 229:1371–1375, 1975.

Cox, R. H. Wave propagation through a Newtonian fluid contained within a thick-walled, viscoelastic tube. *Biophys. J.* 8:691-709, 1968.

Dobrin, P. B. Biaxial anisotrophy of dig cartoid artery: estimation of circumferential elastic modulus. *J. Biomech.* 19:351–358, 1986.

Dobrin, P. B. and Rovick, A. A. Influence of vascular smooth muscle on contractile mechanics and elasticity of arteries. *Am. J. Physiol.* 217:1644–1651, 1969.

Euler, L. *Principes generaux du mouvement des fluides*. History Academy, Berlin, 1775.

Frank, O. Die Grundforn des arterielien Pulses. *Z. Biol.* 37:483–526, 1899.

Frank, O. Die Theorie der Pulswellen. *Z. Biol.* 85:91–130, 1926.

Fry, D.L. and Greenfield, J.C., Jr. Mathematical approach to hemodynamics with particular reference to Womersley's Theory. In: Attinger, E. O. ed., *Pulsatile Blood Flow*, pp. 85-99. McGraw-Hill, New York, 1964.

Geipel P. S. and Li , J. K-J. Time and frequency domain identification of arterial system model parameters. *Proc. 16th NE Bioeng. Conf.*, pp. 75–76, 1990.

Gopalakrishnan, R. *Pulmonary Arterial Tree: Architectural and Functional Design*. Ph.D. dissertation, University of Pennsylvania, Philadelphia, 1977.

Jager, G. N., Westerhof, N., and Noordergraaf, A. Oscillatory flow impedance in electrical analog of arterial system. *Circ. Res.* 16:121–133, 1965.

Iberall, A. S. Anatomy and steady flow characteristics of the arterial system with an introduction to its pulsatile characteristics. *Math. Biosci.* 1:375-395, 1967.

Kenner, T. and Wetterer, E. Experimentelle Untersuchungen uber die Pulsformen und Eigenschwingungen zweiteiliger Schlauchmodellen. *Pflugers Arch. Gesamte Physiol. Mensche. Tiere* 275:594, 1962.

Klip, W. *Velocity and Damping of the Pulse Wave*. Martinus Nijhoff, The Hague, 1962.

Korteweg, D. J. Uber die Fortpflanzungsgeschwindigkeit des Schalles in elastischen Rohren. *Ann. Phys. Chem.* 5:525–537, 1878.

Lamb, H. On the velocity of sound in a tube as affected by the elasticity of the walls. *Manchester Mem.* 42:1–16, 1898.

Lambert, J. W. On the nonlinearities of fluid flow in nonrigid tubes. *J. Franklin Inst.* 266:83, 1958.

Lambossy, P. Aperçu historique et critique sur le probleme de la propagation des sondres dans un liquide compressible enferme dans un tube elastique. *Helv., Physiol. Pharm. Acta* 8:209–227, 1950.

Laskey W. K., Parker, H. G., Ferrari, V. A., Kussmaul, W. G., and Noordergraaf, A. Estimation of total systemic arterial compliance in humans. *J. Appl. Physiol.*, 69:112–119, 1990.

Li, J. K-J. and Zhu, Y. Arterial compliance and its pressure dependence in hypertension and vasodilation. *Angiology, J. Vasc. Dis.* 45:113–117, 1994.

Li, J. K-J., Drzewiecki, G., and Wang, P. R. Compliance of the aorta in acute hypertension. *Proc. 7th. Internat. Conf. Cardiovasc. Syst. Dynamics* 7:1–3, 1986.

Li, J. K-J., Zhu, Y., and Drzewiecki, G. Linear and nonlinear model-based analysis of arterial compliance in hypertension. *Proc. 5th Int. Biomed. Eng. Symp.*, pp. 273–274, 1994.

Li, J. K-J., Melbin, J., Riffle R. A., and Noordergraaf, A. Pulse wave propagation. *Circ. Res.* 49:442–452, 1981.

Li, J. K-J. Time domain resolution of forward and reflected waves in the aorta. *IEEE Trans. Biomed. Eng.* BME-33:783-785, 1986.

Li, J.K-J., Cui, T., and Drzewiecki, G. Nonlinear model of the arterial system incorporating a pressure-dependent compliance. *IEEE Trans. Biomed. Eng.* BME-37:673–678, 1990.

Li, J. K-J. *Arterial System Dynamics*. New York University Press, 1987.

Li, J. K-J. Pressure-derived flow:a new method. *IEEE Trans. Biomed. Eng.* BME-30:244–246, 1983.

Li, J. K-J. *Comparative Cardiovascular Dynamics of Mammals*, CRC Press, New York, 1996.

Li, J. K-J. Feedback effects in heart-arterial system interaction. *Adv. Exp. Med. Biol.* 346:325–333, 1993.

Li, J. K-J., Cui, T., and Drzewiecki, G. Nonlinear model of the arterial system incorporating a pressure-dependent compliance. *IEEE Trans. Biomed. Eng.* BME-37:673–678, 1990.

Ling, S. C. and Atabek, H. B. A nonlinear analysis of pulsatile flow in arteries. *J. Fluid Mech.* 55:493–511, 1972.

Ling, S. C. Atabek, H. B., Letzing, W. G., and Patel, D. J. Nonlinear analysis of aortic flow in living dogs. *Circ. Res.* 33:198–212, 1973.

Liu Z., Brin, K. P., and Yin, F. C. P. Estimation of total arterial compliance:an improved method and evaluation of current methods. *Am. J. Physiol.* 251:H588–600, 1986.

Lucas C. L., Wilcox, B. R., Ha, B., and Henry, G. W. Comparison of time domain algorithms for estimating aortic characteristic impedance in humans. *IEEE Trans. Biomed. Eng.* BME35:62–68, 1988.

McDonald, D. A. *Blood Flow in Arteries*. Arnold, London, 1960, 1974.

Megerman J., Hansson, J. E., Warnock, D. F., et al. Noninvasive measurement of nonlinear arterial elasticity. *Am. J. Physiol.* 250:H181–188, 1986.

Meister J.-J., Tardy, Y., Stergiopulos, N., Hayoz, D., Brunner, H. R., and Etienne, J.-D. Noninvasive method for the assessment of nonlinear elastic properties and stress of forearm arteries in vivo. *J. Hypertens.* 10(suppl.6):S23–S26, 1992.

Melbin, J. and Noordergraaf, A. General solution for flow and stress phenomena in elastic vessels (Navier-Stokes). *Bull. Math. Biol.* 44:29–42, 1982.

Mirsky, I. Wave propagation in a viscous fluid contained in an orthoptropic elastic tube. *Biophys. J.* 7:165–186, 1967.

Moens, A. I. *Die Pulskurve*. Leiden, 1878.

Morgan, G. W. and Kiely, J. P. Wave propagation in a viscous liquid contained in a flexible tube. *J. Acoust. Soc. Am.* 26:323-328, 1954.

Nichols, W. W. and McDonald, D. A. Wave velocity in the proximal aorta. *Med. Biol. Eng.* 10:327–335, 1972.

Noordergraaf, A. *Circulatory System Dynamics.* Academic, New York, 1978.

Noordergraaf, A. Hemodynamics. In: Schwan, H. P., ed., *Biological Engineering,* McGraw-Hill, New York, 1969.

O'Rourke, M. F. Input impedance of the systemic circulation. *Circ. Res.* 20:365–380, 1967.

O'Rourke M. F. and Yaginuma, T. Wave reflections and the arterial pulse. *Arch. Intern. Med.* 144:366–371, 1984.

Peterson L. H., Jensen, R. E., and Parrel, J. Material properties of arteries in vivo. *Circ. Res.* 8:622–639, 1960.

Pollack, G. H., Reddy, R.V., and Noordergraaf, A. Input impedance, wave travel, and reflections in the human pulmonary arterial tree:studies using an electrical analog. *IEEE Trans. Biomed. Eng.* BME-15:151–164, 1968.

Quick, C. M., Li, J. K.-L., O'Hara, D., and Noordergraaf, A. Reconciliation of Windkessel and distributed description of linear arterial system. *Proc. 1st Summer Bioeng. Conf.* 29:469–470, 1995.

Randall O. S., van den Bos, G. C., and Westerhof, N. Systemic compliance:does it play a role in the genesis of essential hypertension ?. *Cardiovasc. Res.* 18:452–462, 1984.

Resal, M. H. Note sur les petits mouvements d'un fluide incompressible dans un tube e l astique. *J. Math. Pures Appl.* 2:342, 1876.

Rideout, V. C. and Dick, D. E. Difference-differential equations for fluid flow in distensible tubes. *IEEE Trans. Biomed. Eng.* 14:171, 1967.

Simon A. C., Levenson, J. A., Chau, N.P., Pithois-Merli, I. Role of arterial compliance in the physiopharmacological approach to human hypertension. *J. Cardiovasc. Pharmacol.* 19(S5):11–20, 1992.

Simon A. C., Safar, M. E., Levenson, J. A., London, G. M., Levy, B. I., and Chau, N. P. An evaluation of large arteries compliance in man. *Am. J. Physiol.* 237:H550–554, 1979.

Spencer, M. P., Okino, H., Denison, A. B., Jr., and Berry, R. L. Electronic and mathematical models of the circulatory system. *Dig. Int. Conf. Med. Electron.* New York, 1961.

Stergiopoulos, N., Young, D. F., and Rogge, T. R. Computer simulation of arterial flow with applications to arterial and aortic stenoses. *J. Biomech.* 25:1477–1488, 1992.

Stergiopulos, N., Meister, J.-J., and Westerhof, N. Simple and accurate way for estimating total and segmental arterial compliance:the pulse pressure method. *Ann. Biomed. Eng.* 22:392–397, 1994.

Taylor, M. G. The input impedance of an assembly of randomly branching elastic tubes. *Biophys. J.* 6:29–51, 1966.

Ting C., Yang, T., Chen, J., Chen, M., and Yin, F. C. P. Arterial hemodynamics in human hypertension. Effects of angiotensin converting enzyme inhibitors. *Hypertens.* 22:839–846, 1993.

Trazzi S., Ravogli, A., Villani, A., Santucciu, C., Giannattasio, C., Cattaneo, B. M., and Mancia, G. Early cardiac and vascular structural changes in subjects with parental hypertension. *J. Hypertens.* 11(suppl. 5):S78–S79, 1993.

Van Brummelen, A. G. W. *Some Digital Computer Applications to Hemodynamics.* Ph.D. dissertation, University of Utrecht, The Netherlands, 1961.

Van den Bos, G. C., Westerhof, N., Eizinga, C., and Sipkema, P. Reflection in the systemic arterial system:effects of aortic and carotid occlusion. *Cardiovasc. Res.* 10:565–573, 1976.

Weber, E. H. Uber die Anwendung der Welienlehre auf die Lehre vom Kreislaufe des Blutes und ins Besondere auf die Pulsiehre. *Ber. Math. Physi, Cl. Konigl. Sachs. Ges. Wiss.*, 1850.

Westerhof, N., Bosman, F., DeVries, C. J., and Noordergraaf, A. Analog studies of the human systemic arterial tree. *J. Biomech.* 2:121–143, 1969.

Wetterer, E. and Kenner, T. *Grundlagen der Dynamik des arteriellen Pulses.* Springer-Verlag, Berlin, 1968.

Witzig, K. *Uber erzwungene Wellenbewegungen zither, inkompressibler Flijssigkeiten in elastischen Rohren.* Ph.D. dissertation, University of Bem, Switzerland, 1914.

Womersley, J. R. Method for the calculation of velocity, rate of flow and viscous drag in arteries when the pressure gradient is known. *J. Physiol.* 127:553–563, 1955.

Womersley, J. R. The mathematical analysis of the arterial circulation in a state of oscillatory motion. *WADC Tech. Rept.* WADC-TR56–614, 1957.

Young, T. Hydraulic investigations. *Phil. Trans.* 98:164–180, 1808.

# 4 Arterial Pulse Transmission Characteristics

## 4.1. Pressure and Flow Waveforms in Large and Small Arteries

Structural and geometric nonuniformities of the arterial tree give rise to differences in observed pressure and flow waveforms in different anatomic locations in the arterial system. Simultaneous recordings of pressure and flow waveforms in different parts of the vascular tree in human and dog have made clear some distinct features as the pulse wave travels away from the heart. First, the pulse pressure (PP) increases and the flow amplitude decreases progressively, though the mean pressure falls very slowly until reaching the arteriolar beds. The fall of mean blood pressure in the arteriolar beds is dramatic. Second, the rate of rise of the pressure wave in early systole increases and the wavefront becomes steeper; that of the flow wave behaves in just the opposite manner. Third, the incisura, or dicrotic notch, casued by pressure fluctuation as a result of an aortic valve closure, is rounded off as the pressure wave propagates toward the periphery, and the diastolic portion of the pressure wave is accentuated. These observations are illustrated in Fig. 4-1. These changes and their explanations are significant in understanding the functional aspects of the arterial system. Consequently, there is considerable diagnostic information that can be derived from the pressure and flow waveforms.

Simultaneously recorded pressure and flow velocity waveforms with catheter-tip electromagnetic flow and pressure sensors, by Mills et al. (1970), along the aorta and in some large arteries in man, are shown in Fig. 4-2. The gross features of the pressure and flow waveforms are similar to those shown in Fig. 4-1 for the dog. In general, pressure and flow waveforms are similar at corresponding anatomic sites among many mammalian species (Li, 1996).

In systole, the left ventricular (LV) pressure develops rapidly during the cardiac isometric contraction period and when it exceeds the aortic pressure (AoP), the ventricular ejection begins. The ventricular outflow is large and rapid at the onset of ejection, then becomes more gradual, and finally declines toward end-systole. At aortic valve closure, there is backflow,

From: *Arterial Circulation: Physical Principles and Clinical Applications*
By: J. K-J. Li © Humana Press Inc., Totowa, NJ

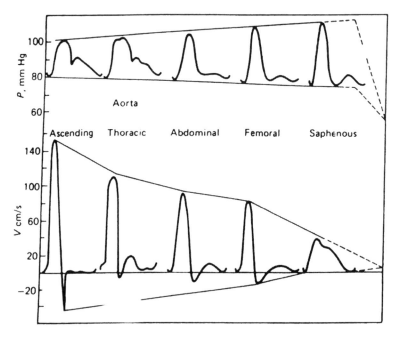

Fig. 4-1. Pressure and flow waveforms in the ascending, thoracic, and abdominal aortas, as well as the femoral and saphenous arteries. Progressive increases in pulse pressure and decreases in pulsatile flow magnitudes are seen. Adapted with permission from McDonald (1960).

followed by small oscillations. In diastole, the aortic flow reaches zero. The diastolic aortic pressure decays precipitously toward end-diastole. In the windkessel approximation, this decay follows a monoexponential pattern. In actuality, there are oscillations superimposed on the diastolic pressure and the decay is not necessarily monoexponential.

The right ventricle and the pulmonary arterial system are known as the low pressure system and the LV and the systemic arterial system are known as the high pressure system. This implies that pulmonary aorta has a much lower pressure amplitude than that of the aorta. The stroke volume is the same, and therefore the flow magnitudes are similar, although their waveforms are quite different. Figure 4-3 obtained by Van den Bos et al. (1982) illustrates the differences. The previous chapter showed that arteries stiffen when pressurized. The pulmonary aorta is much more compliant than the aorta and the pressure waveform tends to be closer in morphology to the flow waveform. This is also because of the less amount of wave reflections in the pulmonary system, which occurs because of the spatial distribution

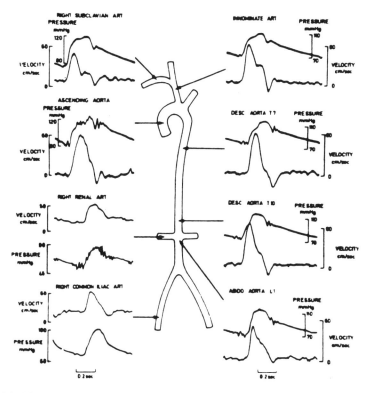

Fig. 4-2. Simultaneously recorded pressure and flow waveforms in different parts of the aorta and in some large arteries in human. Adapted with permission from Mills et al. (1970).

of compliances that are greater in the pulmonary than the higher-pressure, stiffer systemic arteries. From these waveforms, it is also obvious that major reflections do not reach the proximal aortas in early ejection phase. Thus, the time-courses of pressure and flow waveforms are similar during this interval.

With the advent of technology, multisensor catheters capable of simultaneous recordings of several pressure and flow waveforms, are employed. Figure 4-4 illustrates such measurements of pressure waveforms along the aorta (Latham et al. 1985). The advantage of this is in the ease of extracting pulse transmission information, such as pulse wave velocity (PWV) and in the interpretation of hemodynamic alterations in diseased conditions.

The periodicity of the blood pressure waveforms can be seen when a number of consecutive beats are recorded. Figure 4-5 illustrates this with pressure waveforms recorded in the ascending aorta, descending aorta, the abdominal aorta, and the iliac artery, when the catheter-tip pressure trans-

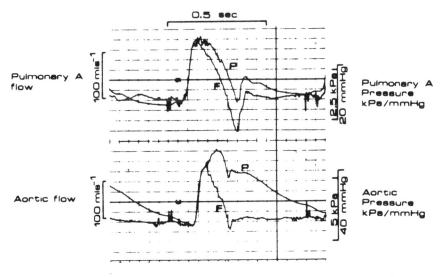

Fig. 4-3. Simultaneously recorded pressure and flow waveforms in the pulmonary aorta (top tracings) and in the ascending aorta (bottom tracings). Notice that the pressure and flow waveforms are more similar in the more compliant pulmonary arterial system. Adapted with permission from Van den Bos et al. (1982).

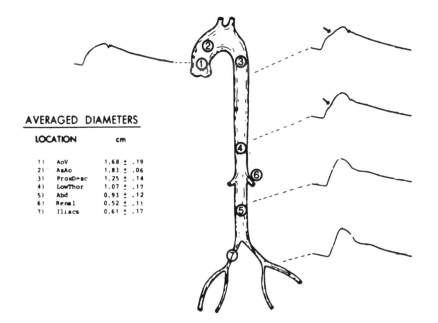

Fig. 4-4. Simultaneously recorded pressure waveforms along the aorta with a multisensor catheter. Corresponding diameters are also shown. Adapted with permission from Latham et al. (1985).

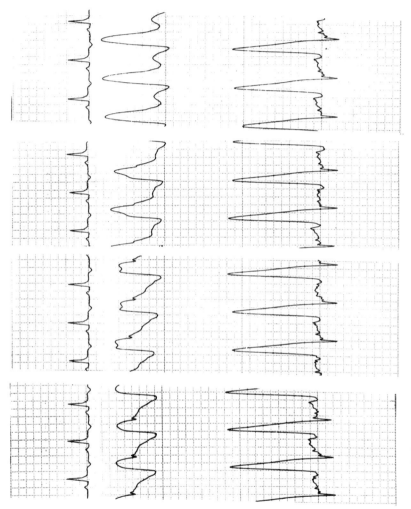

Fig. 4-5. Simultaneously recorded electrocardiogram (top panel), blood pressure (middle panel), and ascending aortic flow (bottom panel) waveforms. Pressure waveforms in the ascending aorta (first left), descending aorta (second left), abdominal aorta (second right) and iliac artery (first right) are shown.

ducer is slowly withdrawn away from the heart. Pulse transit delay and PWV can be easily obtained from this figure. The progressive increases in pulse pressure amplitudes, with increasing systolic pressure and decreasing diastolic pressure can be observed. The electrocardiogram is normally recorded as timing reference and for the calculation of cardiac period. The bottom tracing is the ascending aortic flow measured with an electromagnetic flow probe. The waveforms are reproducible following each heartbeat. This is normally true under steady-state conditions.

The influence of respiration on the pressure waveforms is easily observed when consecutive beats are recorded over a respiratory cycle. The respiratory frequency is much lower than that of heart frequency. There are usually small, but significant changes of the systolic, diastolic and pulse pressure because of respiration. There is a condition of pulsus paradoxus, which occurs when the change in BP is excessive during both inspiration and expiration.

Factors that contribute to the modifications of the arterial pulse waveforms need to be considered in order to understand the morphology of the pulses. The fact that ancient Chinese practitioners were able to detect wrist (radial artery) pulsations which were stronger that those at the neck (carotid artery), already suggested that the more distal the pulse away from the heart, the larger was its amplitude. Spengler (1843), and later Von Kries (1892), pointed out that the amplification of pressure pulses was a result of reflections in the periphery. This was carried over to this century, and the significance of peripheral pressure pulse amplification became the topic of considerable interest decades later, by Hamilton and Dow (1939), Alexander (1953), Porje (1946), Remington and Wood (1956), McDonald (1960), Luchsinger et al. (1964), Attinger et al. (1966b), O'Rourke (1967), Westerhof et al. (1972), and, recently, by Li (1982) and Li et al. (1984b).

It has been suggested that reflection is a closed-end type, with arterioles being the major reflecting site (Westerhof et al., 1972), and that reflections of pressure and flow waves are 180° out of phase. A more detailed discussion of reflection is given in this chapter.

The second factor that influences the pulse waveforms is vascular branching, identified as the geometric nonuniformity discussed in Chapter 2. When pressure and flow waves encounter discontinuities, whether because of tapering, branching, or elastic nonuniformity, reflections will occur and modify the propagating waveform. The branching vascular tree has recently been studied through the use of fractal analysis.

The third influential factor is elastic nonuniformity. The vascular wall becomes progressively stiffer toward the periphery, and accounts for the dispersion of wave velocity and, consequently, reflections.

Finally, the wall and fluid viscosities attenuate the pulse wave. The attenuation, or damping, is greater at higher frequencies. The incisura, for instance, is progressively damped as it propagates. Indeed, when the pulse reaches the femoral artery, the characteristic high-frequency features of the aortic pulse have disappeared. Instead, a smooth waveform is seen. When the pulse reaches the arterioles, it is so damped that its waveform approaches sinusoidal.

Thus, pressure and flow pulses are modified as they travel away from the heart, as the result of wave reflections, geometric nonuniformity, elastic nonuniformity, and damping. The most prominent factor is wave reflection, which is the predominant cause of wave distortion in the arterial system (McDonald, 1960; Noordergraaf, 1978; Li et al., 1984b; Li, 1987).

It is now appropriate to discuss the harmonic contents of the pulse waveforms. Any periodic signal satisfying the Dirichlet conditions (convergence conditions) can be expressed by the Fourier (1882) series. The usefulness of the Fourier series, as Lord Kelvin put it, is as "a mathematical poem." Its use in the cardiovascular system was introduced by Aperia (1940), but was first applied to analyze aortic pressure pulse by Porje (1946).

To use the Fourier series, periodicity and linearity need to be satisfied. Periodicity is often observed, i.e., the heart period is usually invariant from beat to beat during a short interval. Attinger et al. (1966a) analyzed in detail the biological use of the Fourier series, and found that the heart rate (HR) and respiratory cycle only vary by 1–3%, corresponding to a maximum spurious harmonic content of 6%. There was no significant difference in either magnitude and phase of the Fourier coefficients, whether they were obtained over one cardiac cycle chosen at random or over one respiratory cycle. Li (1987) utilized an interpolation method to force the cardiac periods and the beginning and the end of pressure pulses to be identical for different beats (Fig. 4-6). Periodicity and linearity are required to perform Fourier analysis of signals. An interpolation method provided by Li (1987) forces the beginning systolic pressure and the end-diastolic pressure signals to be at the same level. The effects of respiration and small transient changes can be corrected by this method.

Blood pressure waveform can be considered an oscillatory part, with sinusoidal components oscillating at different harmonic frequencies, $n\omega$, and phase, $\phi_n$, superimposed on a mean blood pressure:

$$p(t) = \overline{p} + \sum_{n=1}^{N} p_n \sin(n\omega t + \phi_n) \qquad (4\text{-}1)$$

$$\omega = 2\pi f \qquad (4\text{-}2)$$

where $f$ is in Hz or the number of heartbeats per second. For a man with a resting heartbeat of 60 beats/min, then his fundamental cardiac frequency, with $n = 1$, is

$$f = 60/60 \text{ s} = 1 \text{ Hz} \qquad (4\text{-}3)$$

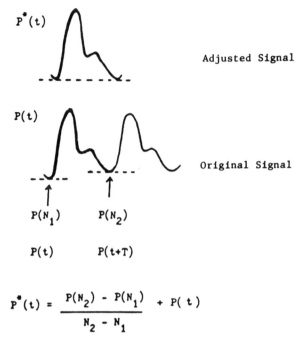

Fig. 4-6. Interpolation method used to adjust pressure signals, in order to apply Fourier analysis more properly.

For the second harmonic, the frequency is, with $n = 2$,

$$f_2 = 2 \times 1 = 2 \text{ Hz} \tag{4-4}$$

and for the fifth harmonic, with $n = 5$,

$$f_5 = 5 \times 1 = 5 \text{ Hz} \tag{4-5}$$

With mild exercise, when the HR increases to 90 beats/min, then the fundamental frequency is no longer at 1 Hz, but rather at $90/60 = 1.5$ Hz. The harmonic magnitudes of a typical aortic pressure pulse and aortic flow pulse are shown in Fig. 4-7. The magnitudes are small and negligible beyond the tenth harmonic component. The Nyquist criterion requires sampling frequency of at least twice the highest-frequency content, in order to reconstruct the original waveform accurately. In the present example, the tenth harmonic would be $1.5 \times 10$, or 15 Hz. The minimal sampling frequency is therefore 30 Hz. In most cases, sampling frequency applied is much higher than this, typically at 100 Hz. In other words, the pressure waveform is digitized at 10 ms intervals.

Luchsinger et al. (1964) have summarized a few criteria pertinent to the linearity of the arterial system discussed in Chapter 3. The first of these

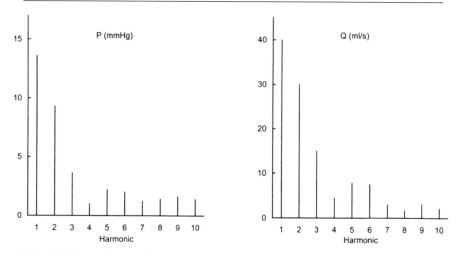

Fig. 4-7. Harmonic magnitudes of a typical aortic pressure pulse and aortic flow pulse.

criteria requires the longitudinal and radial velocities to be small, compared to PWV. In most cases, this is true, except in the aorta, where peak flow velocity may come close to 10% of the wave velocity. The second requires the relative wall displacement to be small, compared with the internal radius, determined by the pressure–radius relationship. This small strain requirement has been shown to be valid by Barnett et al. (1961) and Patel et al. (1963a). The latter requires the diameter to be small, compared with the wavelength, or r<<λ, a popular assumption.

As discussed in Chapter 3, nonlinearities do exist (e.g., Taylor, 1966; Rockwell et al. 1969; Ling et al., 1973), though their magnitude is small and often beyond the capability of recording instruments to register. Nichols and McDonald (1972) found that the arterial system is linear for normal pressure oscillations about the mean value. Linearity was also reported by Dick et al. (1968). In general, linearity is a satisfactory assumption in considering global arterial system behavior.

Measured pressure and flow waveforms contain at most 10 (10× the HR) significant harmonics. In many cases, the accuracy of the harmonics beyond the sixth is subject to uncertainty, because of the noise level and the resolution of the recording instruments. A sampling rate of 100 Hz is adequate for arterial pressure and flow waveforms (Attinger et al., 1966b; Malindzak, 1970). Krovetz et al. (1974) have also analyzed the harmonic contents of intracardiac and arterial pressure waves. Differential pressures and derivatives, however, contain higher-frequency components. Figure 4-8 illustrates the simultaneously recorded pressure and flow waveforms recorded in the ascending aorta of a dog, together with their first derivatives and the ECG. The rate of aortic pressure rise and fall is described by

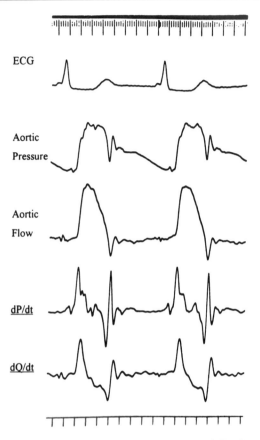

Figure 4-8. Simultaneously recorded electrocardiogram (ECG) of aortic pressure (P), aortic flow (Q), the rate of rise of AoP (dP/dt), and flow acceleration (dQ/dt). Higher frequency contents of the derivatives can be observed.

$dP/dt$. Flow acceleration or the rate of ventricular ejection, is given by $dQ/dt$. The maximum value of aortic flow acceleration, or $dQ/dt_{max}$ has been used as an index of ventricular contractility. It is closely correlated to the maximum rise of LV pressure, or LV $dP/dt_{max}$ The useful information provided by the harmonic analysis of pressure and flow waveforms will be illustrated in the next two subheadings.

### 4.2. Vascular Impedance to Blood Flow

The impedance of the total systemic vascular tree, or the input imped- ance to the arterial system, is defined as the complex ratio by harmonic of pressure to flow. This is so defined when the pressure and flow waveforms are measured at the entrance to the arterial system, namely, at the root or the aorta or ascending aorta. Impedance can also be measured at different parts of the circulation, e.g., when pressure and flow are measured at the femoral artery, then the vascular impedance so obtained represents the impedance of the femoral arterial vascular bed.

Vascular impedance has both a magnitude and a phase for each harmonic. Because pressure and flow are generally not in phase, the impedance possesses a phase angle within ±90°. This is attributed to the time-delayed arrival between the pressure pulse and the flow pulse. When the particular pressure harmonic leads the flow harmonic, then the phase angle between them is positive. Conversely, when the pressure harmonic lags behind the corresponding flow harmonic, then the phase is negative. Phase difference in the frequency domain, therefore, refers to time delay in the time domain.

The relations for the pressure and flow pulse waveforms expressed as magnitude and phase are, for the $n$th harmonic:

$$P_n = |P_n|e^{j(\omega t + \phi_n)} \tag{4-6}$$

$$Q = |Q_n|e^{j(\omega t + \varphi_n)} \tag{4-7}$$

The ratio of pressure to flow is, therefore,

$$\frac{P}{Q} = \frac{|P_n|e^{j(\omega t + \phi_n)}}{|Q_n|e^{j(\omega t + \varphi_n)}} \tag{4-8}$$

The vascular impedance obtained for the $n$th harmonic is, therefore,

$$Z_n = |Z_n|e^{j\Theta_n} \tag{4-9}$$

where the magnitude of impedance is simply the ratio of the pressure amplitude to the flow amplitude for the $n$th harmonic:

$$|Z_n| = \frac{|P_n|}{|Q_n|} \tag{4-10}$$

and the phase lag

$$\Theta_n = \phi_n - \varphi_n \tag{4-11}$$

Pressure and flow waveforms do not necessarily contain the same number of significant harmonics. When the flow harmonic becomes very small, there is a possibility that their ratio or the impedance modulus for that harmonic obtained can be erroneous.

Measurement of the impedance of the vascular bed apparently was first attempted by Randall and Stacy (1956). They, however, did not measure it correctly, nor did they provide a frequency spectrum of the impedance.

Input impedance of the systemic arterial tree was obtained by measuring flow (or computed flow from pressure gradient) and pressure at the ascending aorta in human by several investigators (e.g., Gabe et al. [1964]; Patel et al. [1965]; Mills et al. [1970]; Nichols et al. [1977]; Lasbey et al. [1985]). Numerous investigators also measured it in the dog, including Attinger et al. (1966b), Noble et al. (1967), O'Rourke (1967,1968), O'Rourke and Taylor (1967), Abel (1971), Westerhof et al. (1973), Cox and Pace (1975), Li (1978), Li (1993), and in other mammals (Avolic et al., 1976; Li, 1987) In the pulmonary circulation it has been measured, for example, by Caro and MeDonald (1961), Patel et al. (1963a), Bergel and Milnor (1965), and Reuben et al. (1971). Impedances of certain vascular beds have also been studied (McDonald and Taylor, 1959; McDonald, 1960; Attinger et al., 1966b; O'Rourke & Taylor, 1966; Cox, 1971; and Li, 1978,1982). Figure 4-9 gives an example of the modulus and phase of the vascular impedance measured at the ascending aorta or the input impedance of the systemic arterial tree in normal adults.

In human and dog, the frequency dependence of input impedance resembles that of apparent phase velocity (Subheading 4.3.). The input impedance shows a large decrease in magnitude at very low frequencies (<2 Hz), then oscillates, exhibiting maxima and minima, and eventually reaches a somewhat constant level, low compared to its zero frequency value, at higher frequencies (>5 Hz). The input impedance ($Z$) approaches the characteristic impedance ($Zo$) of the proximal aorta at these high frequencies. The phase of the impedance is initially negative, becoming progressively more positive, and crossing zero at about 3–5 Hz, and remains positive, but close to zero, thereafter.

The large decrease in modulus accompanying a negative phase indicates that the load facing the LV at low frequencies is capacitive in nature; at high frequencies, it is inductive. The inductive and capacitive components must then be equal and opposite, in order to cancel each other out at a frequency at which the phase crosses zero. The viscous losses in the proximal aorta are small, but not negligible elsewhere in the arterial system. Hence, approximating characteristic impedance by the high-frequency values of the input impedance is more accurate in the proximal aorta than in other vessels (Westerhof et al., 1972; Cox and Pace, 1975). Some of these approximations are shown in Table 4-1 (Shi and Li, 1985).

The frequency domain approximation of the characteristic impedance by the average of high-frequency components of the input impedance has been commonly done in the frequency domain:

$$Zo = \overline{Z}(\omega)_{HF} \qquad (4\text{-}12)$$

This is illustrated in Fig. 4-9.

In the time domain, a simple method to approximate characteristic impedance of the aorta is to utilize the fact that, in early ejection, reflected

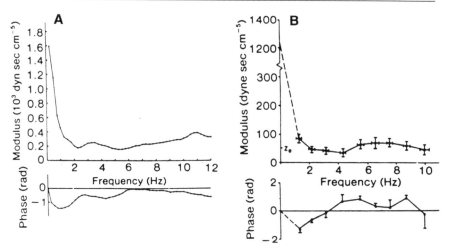

Fig. 4-9. Modulus and phase of the impedance measured at the ascending aorta or input impedance of the systemic arterial tree in a normal adult (**A**) and the average obtained in five adults (**B**). $Z_o$ indicates characteristic impedance of the proximal aorta. Adapted with permission from Nichols et al. (1977).

Table 4-1

Characteristic Impedance of Aorta Estimated from High-Frequency Average of Input Impedance Spectrum

| Authors | Frequency range (Hz) | Estimated $Z_o$ (dyn/s/cm⁵) |
|---|---|---|
| O'Rourke and Taylor (1967) | 15–25 | 230 |
| Abel (1971) | 6–8 | 210 |
| Westerhof et al. (1973) | 3.5–10 | 300 |
| Cox and Pace (1975) | | 270 |
| Clarke et al. (1978) | 1–8 | 180 |
| Peluso et al. (1978) | 1–9 | 288 |
| Dujardin et al. (1980) | 5–10 | 144 |
| Li (1982) | 3–10 | 280 |

waves cannot reach the proximate aorta. In this case, $Z_o$ can be obtained simply from the ratio of instantaneous aortic pressure and flow above their end-diastolic levels (Li, 1986):

$$Z_o = \frac{p(t) - p_d}{Q(t)}$$

(4-13)

This method is valid for the first 60–80 ms of ejection. This is illustrated in Fig. 3-25.

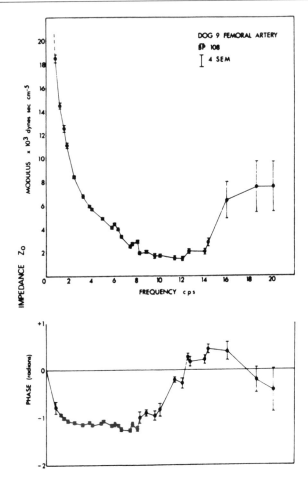

Fig. 4-10. Impedance of the femoral vascular beds obtained by pacing at different frequencies. Adapted with permission from O'Rourke and Taylor (1966).

Another method, also with the assumption that reflected waves do not influence the measurement, is the classic water-hammer formula:

$$Z_o = \frac{\rho c}{\pi r^2} \qquad (4\text{-}14)$$

where $c$ is PWV, $r$ is radius, and $\rho$ is blood density, 1.06 g/cm³. This method can be applied clinically when the cross-section area can be obtained with ultrasound echocardiograph, and the foot-to-foot PWV with a dual-sensor catheter.

Both the input impedance and characteristic impedance moduli increase as the measurement site becomes farther away from the heart. In addition,

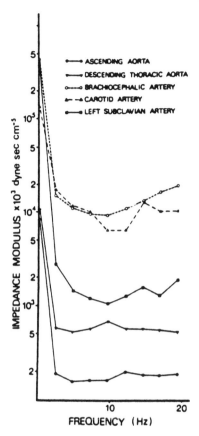

Fig. 4-11. Vascular impedances measured in several systemic arteries at aortic arch. Notice that impedance modulus increases dramatically in smaller arteries. Adapted with permission from Cox and Pace (1975).

zero crossing of the phase occurs at a much higher frequency, as seen in the impedance curves obtained by Patel et al. (1965), O'Rourke and Taylor (1966), and Li (1978) for the femoral bed. Since only harmonic components can appear in the spectrum, extended information can often be obtained by imposing cardiac pacing at different frequencies. An example of this approach is shown in Fig. 4-10. The vascular impedances obtained by Cox and Pace (1975) at aortic arch junction suffice to illustrate these (Fig. 4-11). It is clear from these impedance spectra that the ascending aorta has the lowest impedance modulus and the impedance modulus is higher through the descending thoracic aorta and the left subclavian, the brachiocephalic, and the carotid arteries. The characteristic impedances are also higher in smaller arteries, with their increased stiffness and reduced geometry. Resistance of vascular beds perfused by smaller arteries are also

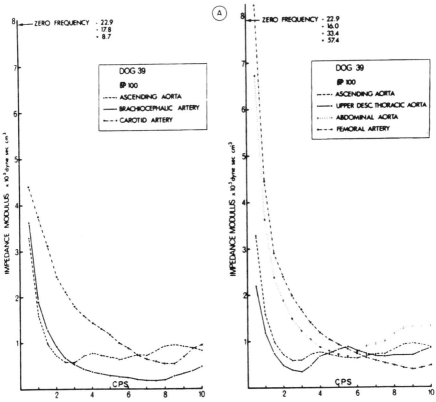

Fig. 4-12. Vascular impedances measured for the upper (left) and lower (right) parts of the body. These information were used in the formulation of the T-tube model of the arterial system. Adapted with permission from O'Rourke (1967).

higher. Vascular impedances obtained from the lower body and upper body arteries by O'Rourke (1967) are shown in Fig. 4-12.

The shape of the input impedance curve is determined by the factors that influence pressure and flow waveforms, as discussed in the previous subheading. But the amount of frequency-dependent reflections dominates the change. The reflection is large and variable, because of the periphery at low frequencies; it is small and constant at high frequencies, because of proximal vessels (Westerhof et al., 1972). The zero frequency component or the total peripheral resistance, $Rs$, is the ratio of mean pressure ($\overline{P}$) to mean flow ($\overline{Q}$). It is significantly higher than the oscillating components. Therefore, the heart appears to be decoupled from peripheral load, so that external cardiac work becomes remarkably independent of HR at high frequencies. It is obvious that the overall input impedance presented to the ventricle, represented by the impedance measured at the ascending aorta, is the lowest among the different vascular beds shown in Figs. 4-11 and 4-12.

In general, input impedance, as predicted by the three-element windkessel model, gives a reasonable overall estimate of experimentally measured input impedance. This is more so in moduli than in phase angles. With vasoconstriction, the impedance modulus is increased, and its minimum is shifted to a higher frequency. With vasodilation, the impedance modulus decreases, and its minimum is shifted to a lower frequency. The manner in which the ventricle responds to changing vascular load has intrigued both investigators and clinicians. The importance in understanding heart–arterial system interaction is dealt with in Chapter 6.

Ventricular afterload is defined as all external factors that oppose ventricular ejection. Arterial input impedance has been suggested as being afterload (McDonald, 1960; Milnor, 1975); however, the interaction of the afterload and inotropic state of the heart still remains unresolved. The energy design of the human circulatory system has been of much interest for many decades (e.g., Evans and Matsuoka, 1915; Rodbard et al., 1959; and Porjé, 1967). The slower the HR, the greater the external work needed to eject a given pulsatile flow (Nichols et al., 1977; Li, 1983). Given a constant impedance spectrum, however, the smaller the pressure and flow generated by the ventricle, the lower the external work. In any case, both the ability of the LV to do work (myocardial performance) and the properties of the arterial system are important in determining the power generated by the ventricle.

The characteristic maxima and minima associated with the input impedance spectrum is closely related to reflections in the arterial system. We have discussed in Subheadings 4.1. and 4.2. how reflections originate, but we need to understand it, not only in a qualitative, but also in a quantitative manner. Both are currently lacking. Wave reflections are dealt with in greater detail in Subheading 4.4.

### *4.3. Pulse Propagation, Wave Velocity, and Damping*

#### 4.3.1. True Pulse Wave Propagation Constant

For a pressure pulse wave propagating along a uniform artery without the influence of wave reflections, the pressures measured simultaneously at any two sites along the vessel are related by:

$$p_2 = p_1 e^{-\gamma z} \tag{4-15}$$

where $p_2$ is the distal pressure and $p_1$ is the proximal pressure, closer to the heart, and $\gamma$ is the propagation constant and $z$ is along the artery in the direction of pulse propagation. The propagation constant obtained under such circumstances is known as the true propagation constant, because it is not influenced by wave reflections. It is a complex variable, and has both magnitude and phase. It is related to the attenuation coefficient, $\alpha$, and the phase constant, $\beta$, by the following:

$$\gamma = \alpha + j\beta \qquad (4\text{-}16)$$

The attenuation coefficient dictates the amount of damping imposed on the propagating pressure pulse due to both viscosity of the blood and viscosity of the arterial walls.

The phase constant arises because of the finite PWV, $c$. In other words, the pressure pulse travels at finite velocity and, therefore, takes a finite amount of time to go through the arterial segment. PWV at any given frequency is given by:

$$c = \frac{\omega}{\beta} \qquad (4\text{-}17)$$

Thus, PWV varies with frequency. This arises, because different pulse waveform harmonic components travel at different velocities. Li et al. (1981) have shown that that true phase velocity increases at low frequencies, and reaches a somewhat constant value at high frequencies, usually beyond the third harmonic.

Experimental measurements of the true propagation constant have met with considerable challenge, since wave reflection arises at numerous locations either along the artery or from proximal and distal vascular beds.

Anliker et al. (1968) utilized high-frequency artificial waves, essentially unaffected by reflections, to obtain phase velocity and attenuation in the dog aorta.

### 4.3.2. FOOT-TO-FOOT VELOCITY

A clinically useful index of pulse wave velocity is the so-called foot-to-foot velocity. Instead of measuring pulse wave velocity at different frequencies, one simply estimates the PWV from the time delay of the onset, or the foot of one pressure pulse to the next. This requires, again, the simultaneous measurements of two pressures separated by a finite distance, $\Delta z$, normally 4–6 cm apart. A double-lumen catheter with two pressure ports connected to two pressure transducers, or a Millar catheter with dual pressure sensors, suffices for such measurement. Thus, the foot-to-foot velocity, $c_f$ is calculated from:

$$cf = \frac{\Delta z}{\Delta t} \qquad (4\text{-}18)$$

where $\Delta z$ is the distance between the two pressure ports or sensors, and $\Delta t$ is the measured time delay. This method assumes that, at the beginning of the pulse or at the start of systole, reflected waves do not yet have sufficient time to arrive to interfere with the propagating pulse.

As an example, referring to Fig. 4-13, the distance between the two pressure measurement sites is 5 cm and the calculated time delay, $\Delta t$, is 60 ms, or 0.06 s, then the foot-to-foot velocity is

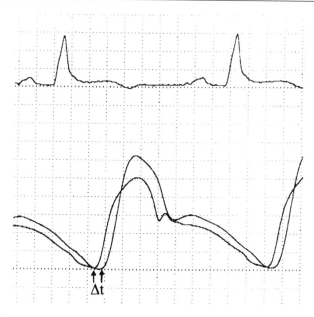

Fig. 4-13. Diagram illustrating how foot-to-foot velocity is calculated, given pressure measurements at different sites separated by a known distance $\Delta z$. Here, the foot-to-foot velocity is given by $c_f = \Delta z/\Delta t$. $\Delta t$ is pulse transit time delay. Notice the peak-to-peak transit time is different from that of the foot-to-foot.

$$c_f = \frac{5}{0.06} = 833 \text{ cm/s or } 8.33 \text{ m/s}$$

(4-19)

Although the peak of the pulse is frequently easier to identify than that at the foot, PWV estimated from the peak, or the peak-to-peak velocity, can show considerable error. This stems from the fact that the peak of the pressure pulse is often contaminated with reflected waves, since it is later in the systole than that at the foot.

With changing geometry and elastic properties away from the ascending aorta, the PWV also changes. Figure 4-14 shows the foot-to-foot velocity measured in different arteries (Nichols and McDonald, 1972). Wave velocity increased from about 5 m/s in the ascending aorta to about 10 m/s in the femoral artery, and higher in the tibial artery.

### 4.3.3. Apparent Propagation Constant and Pressure-Transfer Function

Because of the vascular tree structure and neurohumoral influences, there are considerable differences in the amount of wave reflections that arise in different parts of the circulation. In the presence of reflected waves, one can define an apparent propagation constant where

$$p_2 = p_1 e^{-\gamma_{app} z}$$

(4-20)

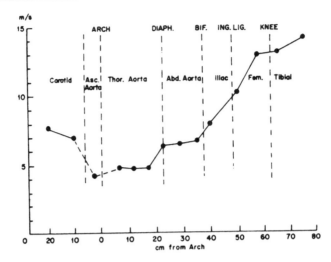

Fig. 4-14. Puse wave velocity recorded as foot-to-foot velocity measured in different arteries. Higher wave velocity in smaller arteries is seen. Adapted with permission from Nichols and McDonald, (1972).

$$\frac{p_2}{p_1} = e^{-\gamma_{app} z} \tag{4-21}$$

and

$$\gamma_{app} = \frac{1}{\Delta z} \ln \frac{p_1}{p_2} \tag{4-22}$$

The apparent propagation constant so defined is dependent on wave reflections and reflect local propagation characteristics. In this case, the separation ($\Delta z$) between $p_2$ and $p_1$ needs to be small, so that it is more representative of the particular artery. When the separation is large, e.g., from the ascending aorta to the abdominal aorta, then the apparent wave velocity obtained may contain branching vessel interactions with their vascular beds. The larger the distance of separation, of course, gives much better accuracy or resolution of the attenuation and phase shift.

In general, the apparent propagation constant at any point along the vessel is defined by:

$$\gamma_{app} = \alpha_{app} + j\beta_{app} \tag{4-23}$$

and $\alpha_{app}$, the apparent attenuation coefficient, is obtained from:

$$\alpha_{app} = \frac{1}{\Delta z} \ln \frac{|p_1|}{|p_2|} \tag{4-24}$$

where $|p_1|$ and $|p_2|$ are the harmonic moduli of $p$, and $p_2$, respectively.

It is clear that $\alpha_{app}$, describes the degree of damping, or the attenuation of the pressure pulse as it propagates between the two arterial sites.

The apparent phase constant, $\beta_{app}$, is obtained from:

$$\beta_{app} = (\phi_1 - \phi_2)/\Delta z \qquad (4\text{-}25)$$

where $\phi_1$ and $\phi_2$ are the harmonic phases of $p$, and $p_2$, respectively. The apparent phase velocity of propagation is calculated from:

$$c_{app} = \frac{\omega}{\beta_{app}} \qquad (4\text{-}26)$$

or, more explicitly,

$$c_{app} = \frac{2\pi f \times \Delta z}{\phi_1 - \phi_2} \qquad (4\text{-}27)$$

$c_{app}$ is also known as the measured velocity. This apparent phase velocity is significantly affected by the presence of wave reflections, in the similar manner as vascular impedance. This, for instance, can be seen from the measurements by Gabe et al. (1964; Fig. 4-15).

The true and apparent propagation constants can be related to characteristic and input impedances as:

$$\frac{\gamma_{app}}{\gamma} = \frac{Z_o}{Z} \qquad (4\text{-}28)$$

This formula also provides a new method for obtaining true propagation constant from measured input impedance and apparent propagation constant (Li, 1978).

Because the apparent phase velocity, $c_{app}$, is influenced by wave reflections in the same manner that input impedance is affected, its frequency spectrum is similar to that of input impedance. Thus, $\gamma_{app}$ is also influenced by wave reflections. An example of the frequency dependence of apparent propagation constant calculated for the femoral arterial bed is shown in Fig. 4-16. These are both dependent on the magnitude and phase of the global reflection coefficient. $\gamma$, on the other hand, is, by definition, independent of reflections, and the manner in which it varies with frequency has been quantified by Li et al. (1980a,1981). It can be deduced that, in the absence of reflected waves, $\Gamma = 0$ and $\beta_{app} = \beta$, i.e., apparent phase velocity equals true phase velocity. This is easily seen in Fig. 4-17, from data obtained by Li et al. (1980a) in a viscoelastic tube. The experimental setup is shown in Fig. 4-18, and was used to determine pulse transmission parameters. This is known as the three-point method for the determination of propagation constant and reflection coefficient, as described in the next subheading.

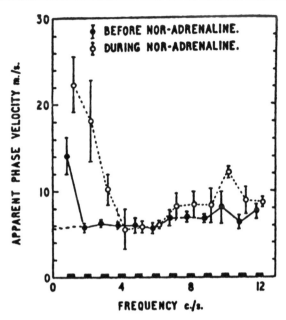

Fig. 4-15. Apparent phase velocity obtained in the aorta during control and noradrenaline infusion. Sharply higher velocity at low frequencies is seen during noradrenaline.
Adapted with permission from Gabe et al. (1964).

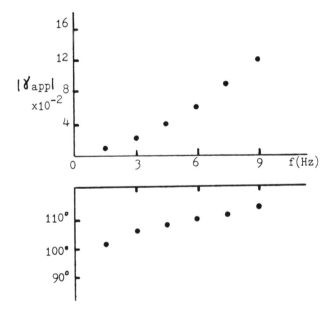

Fig. 4-16. Apparent propagation constant obtained as a function of frequency for the
femoral arterial bed.

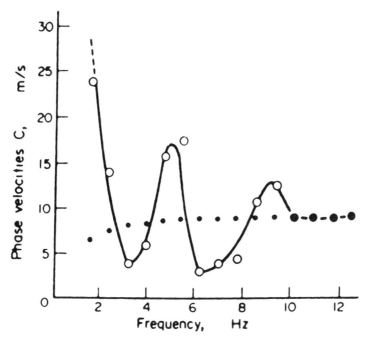

Fig. 4-17. Apparent phase velocity, compared to true phase velocity, in a viscoelastic tube. The influence of wave reflections on apparent phase velocity at low frequencies is clearly seen. At high frequencies the two velocities approach a somewhat constant value.

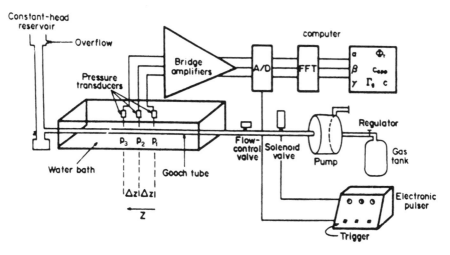

Fig. 4-18. In vitro experimental setup for the determination of pulse transmission parameters (shown on the top-right box) by the three-point method. The three pressures, $p_1$, $p_2$, and $p_3$ are simultaneously measured along the viscoelastic tube. Pulse is generated by the electronic pulser via a solenoid, which also controls the flow rate.

The definition of apparent propagation constant, $\gamma_{app}$, by Eq. 4-22 also represents what is popularly known as the pressure transfer function, or, simply, transfer function. Thus, knowing the transfer function of two arterial sites, one can obtain one blood pressure waveform from the other. This follows from the definition of apparent propagation constant (Eq. 4-20). One can obtain the central aortic pressure waveform from carotid pressure pulse measurement, if the apparent propagation constant or the transfer function is known. This has been demonstrated by Shi et al. (1985). Because carotid pulse, radial pulse, and brachial pulse can be readily obtained noninvasively, this transfer function method has attracted clinical interest in recent years. The goal is to obtain central aortic pressure from noninvasive peripheral arterial pulse measurement. This has recently attempted, for instance, by Karamanoglu et al. (1993). The transfer function obtained takes a form similar to the propagation constant defined above.

### 4.3.4. Methods to Determine the Propagation Constant

Experimental determination of the apparent propagation constant is relatively simpler than that of the true propagation constant. The former can be determined by simultaneously measuring either two pressures (Eq. 4-22) for the pressure pulse, or two flows for the flow pulse. Determination of the true propagation constant, which is independent of wave reflections, in the presence of reflections, however, requires simultaneous measurement of three variables.

Several methods are available to determine the true propagation constant, all of which are based on linear transmission theory. One method utilizes the relations given in Chapter 3, from the definitions of propagation constant as it relates to longitudinal and transverse impedances:

$$\gamma = \sqrt{Z_l/Z_t} \qquad (4\text{-}29)$$

With these relationships, the measurement of pressure and flow, together with their gradients, permit determination of the propagation constant. Cox (1970,1971) applied this method essentially by measuring two pressures a few centimeters apart, a flow midway between them, and the pulsatile change in diameter. Alternatively, the transverse impedance can be obtained from the dynamic pressure–area relationship (Baan, 1970).

If two pressures and flows are measured simultaneously at two sites along a uniform vessel, the propagation constant can be obtained from:

$$\gamma = \frac{1}{\Delta z} \cosh^{-1} \left[ \frac{p_1 Q_1 + p_2 Q_2}{p_2 Q_1 + p_1 Q_2} \right] \qquad (4\text{-}30)$$

where $\Delta z$ denotes the distance between the two sites. Subscript 1 refers to the upstream site; Subscript 2 to the downstream site. This method has been applied by Milnor and Nichols (1975) and Milnor and Bertram (1978).

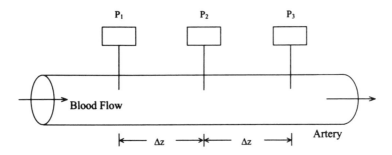

Fig. 4-19. Schematic representation of the three-point method. Pressures $P_1$, $P_2$, and $P_3$, are measured simultaneously at equidistant $\Delta z$ apart.

A vessel occlusion method was investigated by Busse et al. (1979) and Wetterer et al. (1978). The method was first evaluated by Gessner and Bergel (1966).

A fourth method utilizes the simultaneous recording of three pressures along a uniform vessel. The method was suggested by Taylor (1957) and applied later by Gessner and Bergel (1966), McDonald and Gessner (1968), Li et al. (1980a, 1981), and recently by Wells et al. (1998). The propagation constant is obtained as:

$$\gamma = \frac{1}{\Delta z} \cosh^{-1} \left[ \frac{p_1 + p_3}{2p_2} \right] \qquad (4\text{-}31)$$

when differential pressures are measured, $\Delta p_1 = p_1 - p_2$; $\Delta p_3 = p_3 - p_2$. The three pressures, $p_1$, $p_2$, and $p_3$, are simultaneously measured at an equal distance ($\Delta z$) apart. The schematic representation of this three-point method is shown in Fig. 4-19.

### 4.3.5. EXPERIMENTALLY MEASURED PROPAGATION CONSTANT, PHASE VELOCITY, AND ATTENUATION COEFFICIENTS

The three-point pressure method was extensively evaluated by Li et al. (1980a) in a hydrodynamic model. Subsequently, this method was applied to investigate pulse wave propagation in dogs (Li et al., 1981) with respect to contributions by vascular wall elastic and geometric properties, vessel wall and blood viscosity, and nonlinearities in system parameters and in the equations of motion. Discrepancies in results obtained with different experimental methods and theory were discussed and resolved. Measurements were obtained from the abdominal aorta, as well as the carotid, iliac, and femoral arteries of dogs. The components of the propagation constant, i.e., attenuation coefficient and phase velocity, were obtained for each of the vessels investigated (Figs. 4-20 and 4-21). Results were presented along a continuous path of transmission (abdominal aorta, iliac, femoral),

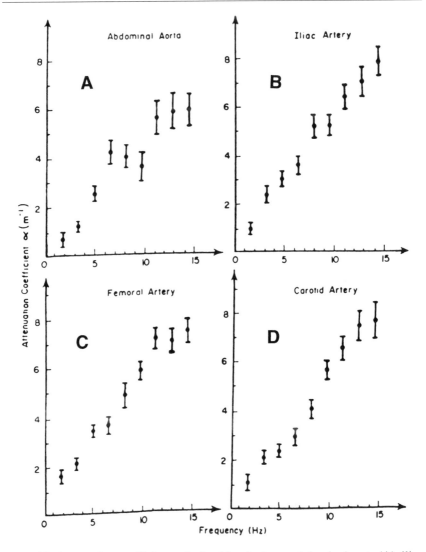

Fig. 4-20. Attenuation coefficients obtained for the lower abdominal aorta (**A**), iliac artery (**B**), femoral artery (**C**), and carotid artery (**D**). Mean ± SEM. Adapted with permission from Li et al. (1981).

and it was shown that variations in phase velocity can be explained entirely by the geometric variation of these vessels. Phase velocities were shown to be frequency-independent at $\geq 4$ Hz; attenuation increases progressively for higher frequencies. Comparison of phase velocities obtained by different investigators using the foot-to-foot method, or the dynamic elastic modulus, or the phase velocity spectrum, are shown in Table 4-2. Pulse

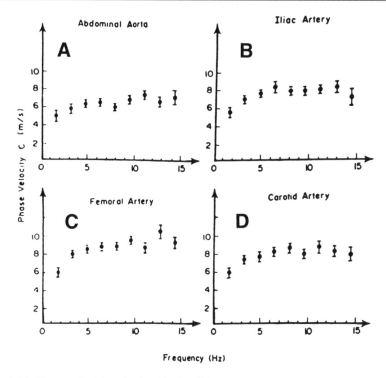

Fig. 4-21. Phase velocities obtained in the **(A)** lower abdominal aorta, **(B)** iliac artery, **(C)** femoral artery, and **(D)** carotid artery. Adapted with permission from Li et al. (1981).

waves travel more slowly in larger vessels, but suffer larger viscous damping in smaller vessels.

Figures 4-22 and 4-23 compare harmonic attenuation obtained by different investigators with different techniques for the carotid and femoral arteries, respectively. Differences in experimental techniques cannot explain these discrepancies. Consideration of geometric taper, nonlinear compliance, all the terms in the equation of motion, and the effect of wall and blood viscosity resolved discrepancies between theoretical models and experimentally derived phenomena. The nonlinear contributions were discussed by Li et al. (1981).

## 4.4. Pulse Wave Reflections and Reflection Sites

Hamilton and Dow (1939) claimed to have observed nodes and antinodes in the pressure pulses and attributed them to the now-famous standing wave phenomena. This standing wave hypothesis to explain pulse amplification was supported by several investigators (Alexander, 1949; Spencer and Denison, 1956). Such an explanation has received a great deal of

Table 4-2
Comparison of Reported Wave Velocities

| Vessel | Velocity (m/s) | Data source | Method | Ref. |
|---|---|---|---|---|
| Abdominal aorta | 6–8 | Dog | f-f[a] | Dow and Hamilton (1939) |
| | 5.5–8.5 | Dog | f-f | Laszt and Müller (1952) |
| | 9.3 | Dog | dE[b], mv[c] | Bergel (1961) |
| | 6.7–7.4 | Dog | f-f | McDonald (1968) |
| | 6.7 | Dog | mv | Li et al. (1981) |
| Iliac artery | 7 | Young men | dE | Learoyd and Taylor (1966) |
| | 8 | Old men | dE | Learoyd and Taylor (1966) |
| | 7-8 | Dog | f-f | McDonald (1968) |
| | 7.7 | Dog | mv | Li et al. (1981) |
| Femoral artery | 8–12 | Dog | f-f | Dow and Hamilton (1939) |
| | 8 | Man | f-f | Kapal et al. (1951) |
| | 8.5–13 | Dog | f-f | Laszt and Müller (1952) |
| | 9.3 | Dog | dE, mv | Bergel (1961) |
| | 18 | Young men | f-f | Learoyd and Taylor (1966) |
| | 13 | Old men | f-f | Learoyd and Taylor (1966) |
| | 8 ± 1.1 | Dog | mv | Gessner and Bergel (1966) |
| | 8.3–10.3 | Dog | f-f | McDonald (1968) |
| | 8.2 | Dog | mv | Cox (1971) |
| | 10.4 ± 0.4 | Dog | dE | Cox (1975) |
| | 8.5 | Dog | mv | Milnor and Nichols (1975) |
| | 8.8 | Dog | mv | Li et al. (1981) |
| Carotid artery | 5–12 | Human | f-f | Bramwell et al. (1922) |
| | 9.4 | Dog | dE, mv | Bergel (1961) |
| | 6.1–7.4 | (Proximal) dog | f-f | McDonald (1968) |
| | 7.7–8 | (Distal) dog | f-f | McDonald (1968) |
| | 8 | Dog | mv | Li et al. (1981) |

[a]f-f, measured as foot-foot velocity.
[b]dE, calculated utilizing dynamic elastic modulus.
[c]mv, mean value from frequency spectrum of phase velocity.

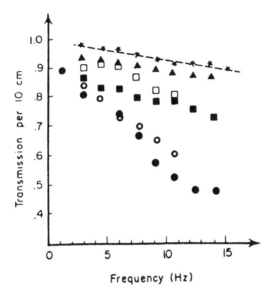

Fig. 4-22. Comparison of damping for the carotid artery plotted as transmission per 10 cm vs frequency. Womersley's theory (dashed line); calculated from Bergel's (1961) in vitro data (closed triangle); McDonald and Gessner (1968), perfused (closed square), in vitro (open circle); in vivo (open square); Wetterer et al. (1978), in vivo (*); Li et al. (1981), in vivo (closed circle). Adapted with permission from Li et al. (1981).

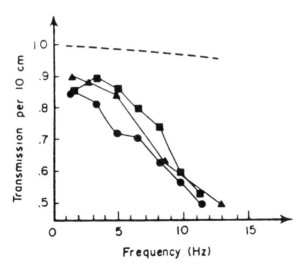

Fig. 4-23. Comparison of damping for the femoral artery, plotted as transmission per 10 cm vs frequency. Womersley's (1957) model (dashed line); Milnor and Nichols (1978), in vivo (closed square); Milnor and Bertram (1978), in vivo (closed triangle); Li et al. (1981), in vivo (closed circle). Adapted with permission from Li et al. (1981).

criticism. Peterson and Gest (1956), for instance, introduced pulses of known, controlled volume into the femoral, iliac, and distal aortic vessels of living dogs, and found that the induced waves became progressively damped and did not reach the aortic root. This led them to reject the standing wave hypothesis, and to conclude that frequency redistribution is an important factor in pulse wave deformation, rather than wave reflections.

Taylor (1957) later demonstrated, by the application of transmission line theory, that, in an attenuating line, no true standing wave can exist. Wiggers (1928), following the approach of Grashey (1881), explained pulse amplification in terms of wave reflection, but without formation of a standing wave. Subsequently, Porje (1946) described, qualitatively, the influence of reflections on the measured wave velocities of harmonics of the aortic pressure pulse. Considerable attention has since been devoted to degrees of reflection and identification of reflection sites in the vascular system, but general agreement has not evolved (Cox and Pace, 1975; Van den Bos et al., 1976; Li, 1978; Murgo et al., 1980,1981; Li et al., 1984b).

Spengler (1843) and Von Kries (1892) were probably the first to point out the amplification of pressure pulses as a result of reflections in the periphery. This mirrors the ancient practitioners' wisdom of feeling palpable pulses for diagnosing the cardiac state. Thus, the pressure and flow pulses contain information about the heart, as well as about the arterial system. Peripheral amplification has also been observed, and became the topic of discussion by Hamilton and Dow (1939), Porje (1946), Remington and Wood (1956), McDonald (1960), Lusinger et al. (1964), O'Rourke (1967), Westerhof et al. (1972), and Li et al. (1982,1984a,1984b).

It has been suggested that reflection is a closed-end type, with arterioles being the major reflection site (also with the greatest fall of mean pressure) and that reflections or pressure and flow waves are 180° out of phase, i.e., an increase in reflected pressure wave causes a decrease in flow amplitude.

The study of pulse waveform contours is important, because of its relevance to many cardiovascular diseases. Alterations in contours are closely related to the mechanical properties of the vessel wall and vascular states, and are linked to hypertension and atherosclerosis (O'Rourke et al., 1970; Safar et al., 1984). In hypertension, for instance, the increased pressure is always associated with increased wave reflections (Li, 1989) and decreased compliance (Simon and Levenson, 1990). Increased wave reflections impede ejection and are detrimental to normal LV function. This increased wave reflection can occur as a consequence of changing vascular bed characteristics or the modification of conduit vessel wall properties.

Pressure (P) and flow (Q) waveforms measured at any site in the arterial circulation can be considered as the summation of a forward, or antegrade, traveling wave and a reflected, or retrograde, traveling wave. We have

$$P = P_f + P_r \qquad (4\text{-}32)$$

$$Q = Q_f + Q_r \qquad (4\text{-}33)$$

It is possible to resolve the measured pressure into forward and reflected pressures, in terms of measured pressure and flow waveforms. The forward wave, or the antegrade (away from the heart) traveling pressure pulse is

$$P_f = (P + Q \cdot Z_o)/2 \qquad (4\text{-}34)$$

Similarly, the reflected pressure wave, or the retrograde (toward the heart) traveling pulse, is

$$P_r = (P - Q \cdot Z_o)/2 \qquad (4\text{-}35)$$

$Z_o$ is the characteristic impedance, defined as the ratio of forward pressure to forward flow, or, in other words, independent of wave reflections, as explained before.

$$Z_o = \frac{P_f}{Q_f} = -\frac{P_r}{Q_r} \qquad (4\text{-}36)$$

$Z_o$ can be obtained from the water-hammer formula, as before:

$$Z_o = \frac{\rho c}{\pi r^2} \qquad (4\text{-}37)$$

where $\rho$ is the density of blood ($1.06$ g/cm$^3$), $c$ is PWV, $\pi r^2$ is the cross-sectional area of the artery.

$Z_o$ can be more easily obtained by the time-domain method (Li, 1986). In essence, peripheral wave reflections do not reach the ascending aorta in early systole. Thus, characteristic impedance can be obtained as the instantaneous ratio of the ascending aortic pressure to flow above the end-diastolic level. This method is illustrated in Fig. 4-24. The instantaneous ratio of aortic pressure to flow is plotted in Fig. 4-25. It can be seen that, in early ejection period, for the first approx 60 ms, this ratio is essentially constant, and equals the characteristic impedance of the proximal aorta (Fig. 4-25).

Similar resolution of flow into its forward and reflected components can be obtained from the set of two equations, and the forward flow is

$$Q_f = (Q + P/Z_o)/2 \qquad (4\text{-}38)$$

Similarly, the reflected flow wave is

$$Q_r = (Q - P/Z_o)/2 \qquad (4\text{-}39)$$

Pressure and flow into their forward and reflected components can therefore be obtained, based on these sets of equations. With the characteristic impedance determined by the time-domain method above, forward and

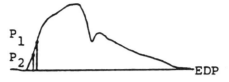

$$Z_o = \frac{P_1 - EDP}{Q_1} = \frac{P_2 - EDP}{Q_2}$$

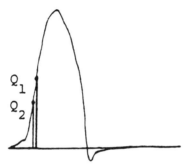

Fig. 4-24. Time-domain method to obtain the characteristic impedance of the ascending aorta from the instantaneous ratio of aortic pressure to flow above the end-diastolic level.

reflected waves can also be resolved in the time domain (Li, 1986). This method of resolving pressure and flow waveforms into their forward and reflected components is simple and fast, and does not require frequency information. Figure 4-26 illustrates the resolved components for both ascending AoP and flow. It can be seen that the retrograde flow has exactly the shape as the reflected pressure wave, but with an opposite sign.

From the above equations, it can be seen that wave reflection has opposite effects on pressure and flow. An increase in wave reflection increases the pressure amplitude, but decreases the flow amplitude. This is particularly evident during different vasoactive states. Figure 4-27 illustrates the waveforms recorded during control, vasoconstriction, and vasodilation conditions. Vasoconstriction is induced by intravenous (iv) infusion of methoxamine, a potent vasoconstrictor. Its primary effect is in increasing peripheral resistance and has little cardiac effect. Vasodilation is induced by iv infusion of nitroprusside, a common vasodilator that can profoundly decrease peripheral resistance and increase arterial compliance. The pres-

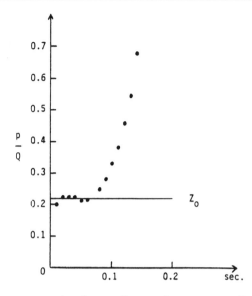

Fig. 4-25. Instantaneous ratio of ascending aortic pressure to flow plotted against time. Pressure and flow were sampled at 10 ms intervals. The ratio is approximately constant for the first 60 ms. The value of the characteristic impedance, $Z_o$, is obtained as shown by the constant line.

sure waveform during strong vasodilation more closely resembles that of the flow waveform.

Figure 4-28 shows ascending AoP (top) and flow (bottom) waveforms, resolved into their respective forward ($P_f$, $Q_f$), or antegrade, and reflected ($P_r$, $Q_r$), or retrograde, components. It is clear that wave reflection exerts opposite effects on pressure and flow waveforms. The increased reflected pressure component adds to the forward wave to result in the measured pressure waveform. Reflected wave has a more significant role in mid- to late systole. Time from the onset of the pressure wave to the peak of peak forward wave is relatively short and significantly earlier than the time to reach the peak of reflected component. Wave reflection decreases the flow, because the reflected component of flow is mostly negative. With an increased amount of wave reflection, pressure amplitude is increased, which is seen in the case of strong vasoconstriction shown in Fig. 4-29 in which reflected waves arrive earlier and with greater magnitudes. As a consequence, the pulse pressure is significantly increased, with a concurrent decrease in flow amplitude. The time needed for forward pressure to reach its peak is not too different from that of the reflected component. With profound vasodilation (Fig. 4-30), the measured pressure and flow waveforms resemble each other, and both peak at about the same time. The

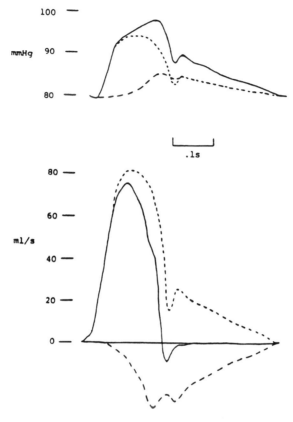

Fig. 4-26. Time-domain-resolved forward and reflected pressure and flow waveforms. The reflected components of pressure and flow have opposite sign.

reflected wave is almost abolished.; thus, both pressure and flow waves are transmitted with maximal efficiency.

The amount of the forward-traveling pressure pulse that is reflected can be expressed as the harmonic ratio of reflected wave to the forward wave in the frequency domain. This defines the reflection coefficient:

$$\Gamma = \frac{P_r}{P_f} \qquad (4\text{-}40)$$

Reflection coefficient has both a modulus and a phase, and hence is a function of frequency:

$$\Gamma = |\Gamma| \angle \phi_\Gamma \qquad (4\text{-}41)$$

Reflection coefficients calculated for the normal, vasoconstricted, and vasodilated conditions obtained in several experiments are shown

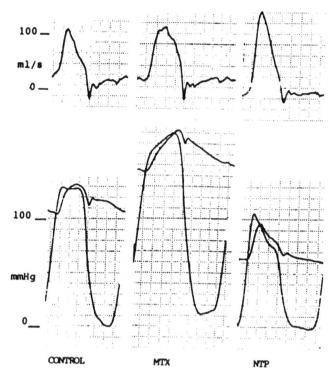

Fig. 4-27. Simultaneously recorded pressure and flow waveforms during control (left), methoxamaine-induced vasoconstriction (middle), and nitroprusside-induced vasodilation (right).

in Fig. 4-31. For the fundamental harmonic, the mean value of the reflection coefficient at control is about 0.45. This is increased to 0.65 during vasoconstriction, and decreased to about 0.15 during vasodilation. The reflection coefficient remains low for higher frequencies during vasodilation.

### 4.4.1. THE REFLECTION COEFFICIENTS

As noted in Subheading 4.2., use of the impedance concept has been extensive. It has been applied to calculate the magnitude of the reflection coefficient ,and to predict reflecting sites. It is well known in the field of transmission engineering that, if the characteristic impedance, load reflection coefficient, and propagation constant are given, the transmission line can be completely defined. This idea has been applied by several investigators (e.g., Taylor, 1957; Westerhof et al., 1969).

For a single uniform line with characteristic impedance, $Z_o$, and terminated with load impedance, $Z$, the reflection coefficient, $\Gamma$, is given by:

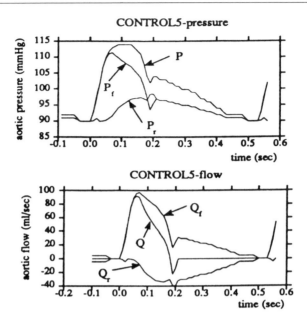

Fig. 4-28. Ascending AoP (top) and flow (bottom) waveforms resolved into their respective forward ($P_f$, $Q_f$), or antegrade, and reflected ($P_r$, $Q_r$), or retrograde components. Notice that wave reflection exerts opposite effects on pressure and flow waveforms, as seen from $Q_r$ and $P_r$. Provided by Y. Zhu.

$$\Gamma = \frac{Z - Z_o}{Z + Z_o} \qquad (4\text{-}42)$$

The reflection coefficient so obtained is therefore a complex quantity, with modulus $\Gamma$ and phase $\phi_\Gamma$ varying with frequency. For the arterial system, $Z_o$ is identified as the characteristic impedance of the ascending aorta. $Z$ is the input impedance of the systemic arterial tree. Thus, the global reflection coefficient does not differentiate its individual contributing sources. Global reflection coefficient for the arterial tree obtained by Westerhof et al. (1972) calculated by this approach is shown in Fig. 4-32.

Westerhof et al. (1969) made a condensed comparison of other models to their analog of the human systemic arterial tree, and observed that, for frequencies of 1 and 5 Hz, the local reflection coefficients are small and relatively independent of frequency, as concluded theoretically by Wormersley (1958). Addition of viscous damping of the wall did not affect the phase of $\Gamma$. Li et al. (1984a,1984b) discussed the directional sensitivity of wave reflections. Experimental results show that vascular branching is well matched in normal physiological conditions. Data from Li et al. (1984b) demonstrate this. Characteristic impedances were computed from

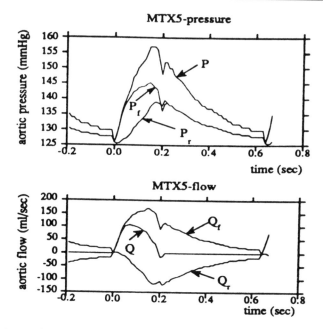

Fig. 4-29. Ascending AoP and flow waveforms resolved into their respective forward and reflected components during vasoconstriction induced by iv infusion of methoxamine. Notice the significantly increased reflected pressure component.

the water-hammer formula: The backward (toward the heart) reflection coefficient is much larger than the forward one at vascular branching, indicating a larger mismatch, and that the reflection is directional.

Model studies show that, unlike local reflection coefficients, global reflection coefficients are strongly frequency-dependent, both in amplitude and in phase, which were appreciably altered when viscous damping of the wall was introduced. Experimental data obtained by Westerhof et al. (1972), utilizing Eq. 4-42, assuming $Z_o$ equals the high-frequency average of $Z$, show a precipitous decrease in the magnitude of reflection with increasing frequency (Fig. 4-32). As expected, vasoconstriction increased, and vasodilation decreased, wave reflections. One must distinguish between reflection at vascular branching of large vessels and reflections at the arteriolar part of the system. The former contributes only a small and somewhat constant portion to the returning wave; the latter exerts a variably large amount.

Li et al. (1984b) utilized the three-point pressure method (Li et al., 1980a, 1981) to measure the amount of reflections arising from the femoral arterial bed. The global reflection coefficient ($\Gamma$) is defined as the ratio of retrograde pressure to antegrade pressure pulses, i.e.: in which $|\Gamma|$ and $\phi_\Gamma$ denote magnitude and phase of $\Gamma$, respectively.

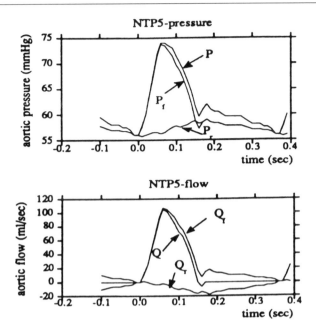

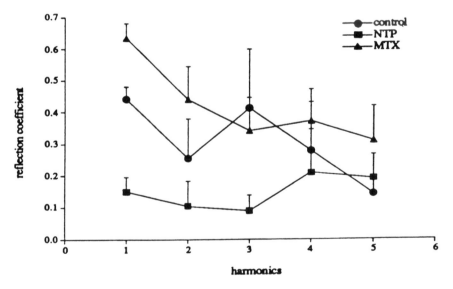

Fig. 4-30. Ascending AoP and flow waveforms resolved into their respective forward and reflected components during vasodilation induced by iv infusion of nitroprusside. Notice the similarity between the pressure and flow waveforms, and that the reflected components are small.

Fig. 4-31. Global reflection coefficients obtained during control (circle), vasoconstriction (triangle), and vasodilation (square) conditions.

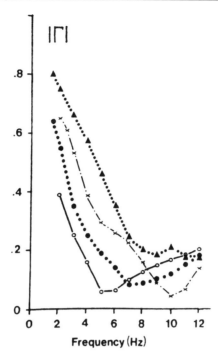

Fig. 4-32. Global reflection coefficients of the systemic arterial tree plotted as a function of frequency during control (closed circle), vasoconstriction (x), vasodilation (open circle), and aortic occlusion (triangle). Magnitudes of reflection coefficients are small and variable at high frequencies. Adapted with permission from Westerhof et al. (1972).

$$\Gamma = P_r/P_f = \ |\Gamma|e^{j\phi_\Gamma} \qquad\qquad (4\text{-}43)$$

Figure 4-33 illustrates pressure waveforms from the femoral artery for control (A), vasodilated (B), and vasoconstricted (C) states. Compared to the control data, a steepened wavefront is observed during vasoconstriction, i.e., a more rapid systolic pressure rise, with a shortened systolic interval, higher peak systolic and pulse pressures, and a distinct dicrotic wave. Mean pressure increased by about 40 mmHg. With strong vasodilation, a slower systolic pressure rise is observed, as well as a lengthened systolic interval, lowered peak systolic and pulse pressures, and abolishment of the dicrotic wave. Mean pressure decreased by about 30 mmHg. The corresponding pressure waveforms, recorded during control, vasodilation with acetylcholine, and vasoconstriction with norepinephrine, are shown in this figure. Notice that the diastolic pressure wave is abolished during acetylcholine-induced vasodilation. The diastolic wave is accentuated during norepinephrine induced vasoconstriction.

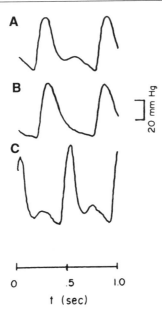

Fig. 4-33. Pressure waveforms measured in the femoral artery during control (**A**), acetylcholine-induced vasodilated (**B**), and norepinephrine-induced vasoconstricted (**C**) states. Adapted with permission from Li et al. (1984b).

Reflection coefficients for an isolated vascular bed, such as the femoral arterial bed obtained by Li et al. (1984b) is shown in Fig. 4-34. These were obtained by the three-point pressure methods applied to isolated femoral arterial segments. For control data (circle), the magnitude of the reflection coefficient ranged from 0.42, at 1.6 Hz, to 0.22, at 9.6 Hz. vasoconstriction coefficient, to about 0.65 at 1.6 Hz and 0.32 at 9.6 Hz. Vasodilation (triangles) decreased the reflection coefficient to a value less than 0.1 for all frequencies. These data and those of O'Rourke and Taylor (1966) show that alterations in vascular impedance of this bed can be attributed to alterations of reflection coefficients caused by such vasoactive agents. A variable degree of vessel occlusion can also appreciably alter the reflection coefficients and the shapes of pulse pressure and flow (Westerhof et al., 1973; Van den Bos et al., 1976). Forward and reflected waves have also been investigated by Caro et al. (1967), Sperling et al. (1975), and Newman et al. (1979).

### 4.4.2. BLOOD PRESSURE AUGMENTATION INDEX

A simplified approach of interpretation to the effect of wave reflection in the augmentation of aortic pressure pulse was introduced by Murgo et al. (1980), and is illustrated in Fig. 4-35. Ascending AoP waveforms are

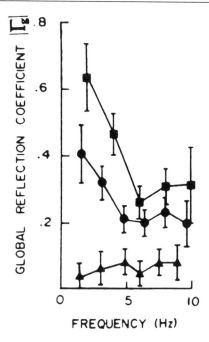

Fig. 4-34. Reflections arising from the femoral vascular bed during control (circle), vasoconstriction (square), and vasodilation (triangle). Reflection coefficients were computed from the three-point method. Adapted with permission from Li et al. (1984b).

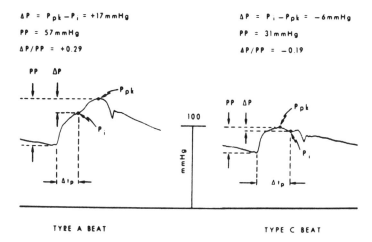

Fig. 4-35. Aortic pressure waveforms, illustrating the three types of waveform configurations, defined as type A, type B (similar to A, but $AI < 0.12$), and type C beats. The augmentation index is defined as $\Delta P/PP$. $P_s$ ($P_{pk}$), $P_d$, $P_i$, and $PP$ are peak systolic, diastolic, inflection, and pulse pressures, respectively. Adapted with permission from Murgo et al. (1980).

defined in terms of their morphological differences, and are separated into type A, type B, and type C configurations. Peak systolic pressure ($P_s$ or $P_{pk}$), diastolic pressure ($P_d$), PP, pressure at inflection point ($P_i$) and the augmented pressure, $\Delta P$, are defined. Systolic pressure augmentation is given by

$$\Delta P = P_s - P_i \qquad (4\text{-}44)$$

and the corresponding augmentation index is given by

$$AI = \frac{\Delta P}{PP} = \frac{P_s - P_i}{P_s - P_d} \qquad (4\text{-}45)$$

Type A waveform is defined when the peak systolic pressure occurs in late systole, after an inflection point, and the augmentation index is greater than 0.12. Type B is similar to A, except the augmentation index is less than 0.12. In type C configuration, peak systolic pressure occurs prior to the inflection point and the augmentation index is negative. Figure 4-36 illustrates augmentation index that can be obtained during transient changes in pressure waveforms caused by bilateral occlusion of the femoral artery by external compression. The calculated augmentation indices for the two beats are

$$AI = \frac{\Delta P}{PP} = \frac{10}{60} = 0.167 \qquad (4\text{-}46)$$

and

$$AI = \frac{\Delta P}{PP} = \frac{20}{70} = 0.286 \qquad (4\text{-}47)$$

Thus, the augmentation index can vary from beat to beat.

Input impedance spectra obtained for the three types of AoP configurations are shown in Fig. 4-37. Differences in total peripheral resistance and characteristic impedance are easily seen. Oscillations in impedance maxima and minima can also be observed. Thus, the three types of waveforms represent different vascular states.

The augmentation index should be used with caution in interpreting overall effects of wave reflection. Although this index has been used to represent reflection ratio, it really is not equivalent to the reflection coefficient in the forgoing discussions. Augmentation index is merely a single number, and does not represent the frequency dispersion and content of the reflected wave. In addition, changing ventricular or cardiac state, i.e., contractility, can also alter the augmentation index.

### 4.4.3. REFLECTION SITES

Wave reflection sites exist all over the systemic arterial tree, as the result of geometric and elastic nonuniformities, branching, and impedance mis-

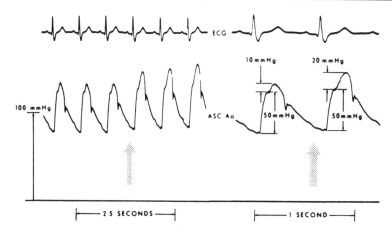

Fig. 4-36. Augmentation index that can be obtained during transient changes in pressure waveforms because of bilateral external compression of the femoral artery. Adapted with permission from Murgo et al. (1980).

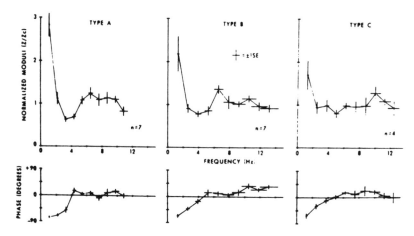

Fig. 4-37. Input impedance spectra obtained for the three types of aortic pressure configurations. Different spectral contents result in differences in impedance modulus and phase angles. Adapted with permission from Murgo et al. (1980)

matching at arterial terminations. Therefore, reflections cannot originate from one site only. Indeed, there is no agreement on the location of reflecting sites (O'Rourke, 1967). McDonald (1960) and Remington (1963) have shown that the major reflection site, as seen from the proximal aorta, appears to be in the region of the pelvis. Arndt et al. (1971), however, stated that the first major potential reflecting site is at the branching of the brachiocephalic artery from the aorta. O'Rourke (1967) stated that the aortic valve appears to be relatively unimportant in arterial reflection phenomena, which is in disagreement with McDonald (1974) and Arndt et al. (1971). His T-model does not take into account nonuniformities, nor the frequency dependence of wave reflection, though it is useful in comparative hemodynamics (*see* Chapter 7).

Arndt et al. (1971) concluded that the aortic arch and the descending thoracic aorta are not effective reflecting sites (Cox, 1975), and suggested the arteriolar beds near the heart as a possible site for late systolic reflections. A decrease in the reflection coefficient with increasing pressure was also observed.

Although there is no major agreement on the reflecting sites, the arterioles are recognized as the principal sites for wave reflection (McDonald, 1960; O'Rourke and Taylor, 1966; Westerhof et al., 1972), and the reflection coefficient as being high (O'Rourke, 1967; Westerhof et al., 1972). Some models, however, assumed lower peripheral reflections (Wetterer and Kenner, 1968).

Reflection sites have generally been determined from the first impedance minimum, and subsequent calculation:

$$\lambda_{min} = \frac{c}{f_{min}}$$

(4-48)

and

$$L_R = \frac{\lambda_{min}}{4}$$

(4-49)

$\lambda_{min}$ and $f_{min}$ are the wavelength and frequency corresponding to the impedance minimum. $L_R$ is the distance of the effective reflection site from the point of measurement.

The representation of the magnitudes of reflection coefficient in the time domain can provide an easy means to differentiate the amount of wave reflections arriving at different intervals in systole. In addition, the effective reflection sites can be readily calculated, as demonstrated by Lei et al. (1996), and shown in Fig. 4-38. Reflection is larger and arrives earlier in systole during vasoconstriction, but is greatly reduced in vasodilation. Notice the periodicity in the reflection coefficient.

### 4.5. Pulse Transmission at Vascular Branching

A local reflection coefficient can be defined for vascular branching only:

$$\Gamma_l = \frac{Z_{o1} - Z_{o2}}{Z_{o1} + Z_{o2}}$$

(4-50)

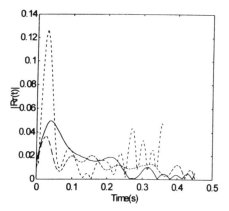

Fig. 4-38. Time domain interpretation of the reflection coefficient. Distances to reflection sites can be calculated from the peak-to-peak time intervals. Control (solid line), vasoconstriction (dotted line), and vasodilation (dashed line).

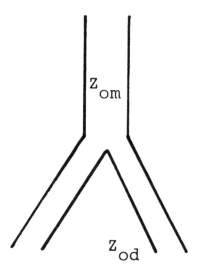

Fig. 4-39. Diagrammatic representation of a branching vascular junction. An equibifurcation is illustrated with characteristic impedance of the mother ($Z_{om}$) and daughter ($Z_{od}$) vessels, respectively.

where $Z_{o1}$ represents the resultant parallel combination of the characteristic impedance of branching daughter vessels, and $Z_{o2}$ is the mother vessel's characteristic impedance. For an equibifurcation (Fig. 4-39), one obtains:

$$\Gamma_l = \frac{Z_{od} - Z_{om}}{Z_{od} + Z_{om}} \qquad (4\text{-}51)$$

$$\Gamma_l = \frac{Z_{od} - 2Z_{om}}{Z_{od} + 2Z_{om}}$$

(4-52)

### 4.5.1. Area Ratio Concept

Karreman (1952) used the concept of area ratio in studying wave reflection at the arterial junction. By assuming that both the wall and fluid are nonviscous, and that wall thickness remains the same for an infinitely long tube, he arrived at a value of area ratio (the ratio of the sum of the areas of daughter vessels to that of the mother vessel), for a reflectionless bifurcation of about 1.15.

Womersley (1958) later arrived at a similar result, with a correcting factor, $q$, for a tethered elastic tube containing viscous liquid, with the assumption that the daughter vessels have identical characteristics ($r_d$, $c_d$):

$$\lambda' = 2(r_d/r_m)^2 \times (c_m/c_d) \times q$$

(4-53)

The local reflection coefficient is then given by:

$$\Gamma_l = \frac{1 - \lambda'}{1 + \lambda'}$$

(4-54)

Exact matching is not possible (perfect matching is only obtained when $\alpha_\omega \to \infty$), though the minimum reflection is only a few percent. This is shown in Fig. 4-40. The area ratios for the aortic junctions are usually between 1.15 and 1.25, which represent a very small number of reflections (Li et al., 1984a,1984b). These same small local reflection coefficients were found on the analog by Westerhof et al. (1969). For optimum energy transfer, the area ratio needs to be close to one (Sarpkaya, 1967; Hunt, 1969; Caro et al., 1971). Tables 4-3 and 4-4 further emphasize this.

The area ratio concept has received continued attention (Li, 1985). Its practical applications have been demonstrated by Gosling and Newman (1971). Area ratio is clinically measured by injecting radiopaque dye to obtain radiographs, and by assuming a circular crosssection (Fig. 4-41), as suggested by Fry et al. (1964), for the junction vessels. Newman and Bowden's (1973) experimental result (minimum reflection when area ratio equals 1.23) conformed closely to that given by Womersley's theory (minimum reflection when area ratio equals 1.26) for the equibifurcation.

In small muscular vessels, viscous damping is appreciably more important than in large vessels. In these vessels, the point of minimum reflection (in the reflection vs area ratio plot) is shifted to a larger area ratio, accompanied by a larger phase change.

The importance of topological geometry (Zamir, 1982) and elastic properties at vascular branching junctions can be easily appreciated from the

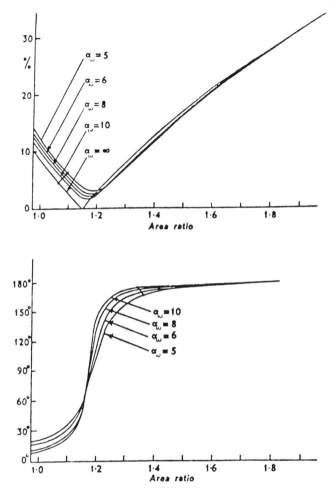

Fig. 4-40. Reflections at vascular branching. Local reflection coefficients computed for an equibifurcation are plotted against area ratios. Adapted with permission from Womersley (1958).

measurement of local reflection coefficients involving characteristic impedances of junction vessels (Li, 1986b). Figure 4-42 shows that the local reflection coefficient is significantly increased when the vessel lumen radius is progressively decreased downstream from the junction (daughter vessels). But when the branching vessels become stiffer with increased elastic modulus, such changes in local reflection coefficient arer moderate (Fig. 4-43). This indicates that junction geometry is more dominant in determining pulse transmission through vascular branching than elastic factors (Li, 1986b).

Table 4-3
Local Reflection Coefficients ($\Gamma_l$) and Area Ratios at Aortoiliac Function

| Dog | $\Gamma_{ls^*\to b}$ | $\Gamma_{lb^*\to s}$ | $\Gamma_{ls\to b}$ | $\Gamma_{lb\to s}$ |
|---|---|---|---|---|
| 1 | 0.37 | −0.68 | 0.11 | −0.74 |
| 2 | 0.32 | −0.66 | 0.06 | −0.73 |
| 3 | 0.30 | −0.65 | 0.04 | −0.72 |
| 4 | 0.36 | −0.68 | 0.10 | −0.74 |
| 5 | 0.28 | −0.68 | 0.01 | −0.76 |
| 6 | 0.35 | −0.66 | 0.09 | −0.74 |
| Average | 0.33 | −0.67 | 0.07 | −0.74 |
| ±σ(SD) | −0.036 | −0.018 | ±0.039 | ±0.013 |
| $\Gamma_l$, as predicted by areas only | 0.29 | −0.64 | −0.02 | −0.73 |

s, source; b, branch. *Continuation of abdominal aorta occluded at iliac bifurcation.

Table 4-4
Aortic Arch Local Reflection Coefficients

| | Local reflection | Crosssectional area ratios (b/s) |
|---|---|---|
| AA → (DTA, LSA, BCA) | 0.04 | 1.08 |
| DTA → (AA, LSA, BCA) | −0.35 | 2.00 |
| BCA → (AA, LSA, DTA) | −0.83 | 8.69 |
| LSA → (AA, BCA, DTA) | −0.87 | 11.17 |
| DTA → (BCA, LSA, AA occluded) | 0.37 | 0.56 |
| | calculated from $Z_s$, $Z_b$ | |

AA = Ascending aorta, DTA = descending thoracic aorta, LSA = left subclavian artery, BCA = brachiocephalic artery.

## 4.6. Pulse Transmission to Vascular Beds

### 4.6.1. Pressure and Flow Waveforms in Arterioles and Capillaries

Pulses, originating at the left ventricle, are modified as they propagate toward the periphery. This is attributed to the effects of blood viscosity, to arterial viscoelasticity resulting in frequency dispersion and selective attenuation, and to site-dependent summation of incident and reflected pulses. Pulsations, however, persist even in the microcirculation.

Quantification of peripheral resistance has long been of interest to both researchers and clinicians. Since the largest mean pressure drop occurs in the arteriolar beds, these latter have been shown to contribute mostly to the peripheral resistance (Li, 1987).

It has been presumed for decades that flow in the microcirculation, particularly in the arterioles and capillaries, is entirely steady flow. Con-

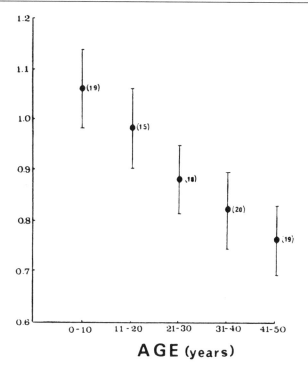

Fig. 4-41. Area ratios obtained from angiographic recording of the human aortoiliac bifurcation plotted against each decade of age. Area ratios decrease significantly with increasing age. Adapted with permission from Gosling et al. (1971).

sequently, Poiseuille's formula has been applied. Poiseuille in 1841 arrived at an empirical relationship relating pressure drop, $\Delta P$, to steady flow $(\overline{Q})$, in a cylindrical vessel with diameter, $D$, and length, $l$.

Thus, the amount of steady flow through a blood vessel is proportional to the pressure drop and the fourth power of the diameter. Independently, Hagen in 1939 had performed numerous experiments, and, at about the same time, arrived at a similar expression. This formula was later modified to the presently known Hagen-Poiseuille equation, or simply, Poiseuille's law:

$$\overline{Q} = \frac{\pi r^4}{8\eta l} \, \Delta p \qquad (4\text{-}55)$$

Although credit has been given fully to Poiseuille, it was Hagenbach in 1860 who found an exact relation between steady flow and fluid viscosity, $\eta$, and the pressure gradient,

$$Q = -\frac{\pi r^4}{8\eta} \frac{dp}{dz} \qquad (4\text{-}56)$$

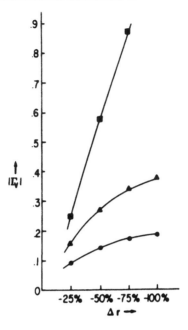

Fig. 4-42. Local reflection coefficient is plotted against the reduction in radius. Sharply increased reflection coefficient is associated with narrowing branching vessel lumen radius.

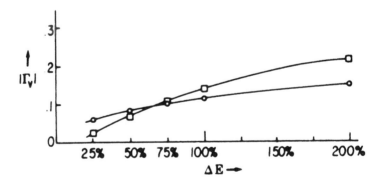

Fig. 4-43. Local reflection coefficient is plotted against the reduction in elastic modulus. Reflection is increased with increased branching vessel stiffness, but the increase is less pronounced, compared with corresponding percentage reduction in lumen radius.

Pressure gradient in the Poiseuille's law is simply $\Delta P/l$. Poiseuille resistance to steady flow is, therefore:

$$R_s = \frac{\pi r^4}{8\eta l} \tag{4-57}$$

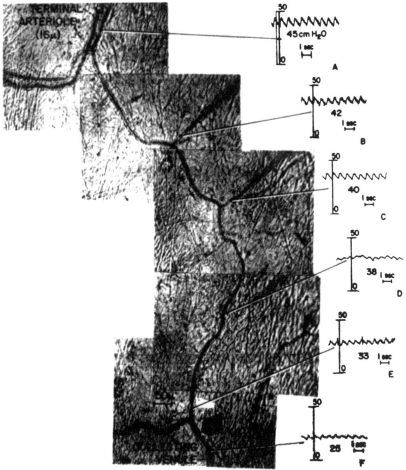

Fig. 4-44. Photomicrographic reconstruction of the microcirculation including the perfusing arterioles, the capillaries and the collecting venules. Direct pulsatile pressure recordings are shown. Adapted with permission from Zweifach (1974).

Steady flow was assumed because of the belief that small peripheral vessels are resistance vessels, preventing pulsations from occurring.

As mentioned above, the largest mean pressure drop occurs in small arterioles. Referring to Chapter 2 regarding the structure of the vascular walls, we see that this is also where smooth muscle tends to exert its influence. Thus, accompanying the smooth muscle (Somlyo and Somlyo, 1968) activation, is a change in vessel lumen radius. Because flow varies by the fourth power of radius, a small change in radius can amount to a large alteration in flow. Thus, the peripheral resistance can alter central arterial flow, and hence cardiac output.

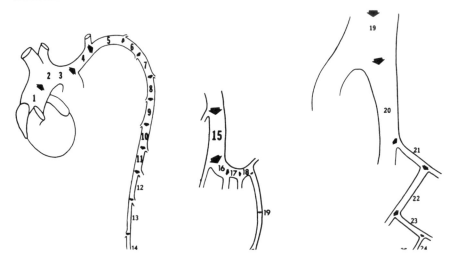

Fig. 4-45. Schematic illustration of the pulse transmission path from the ascending aorta to the index finger artery.

It is now known that pulsatile ejection by the ventricle requires only about 10% additional energy for the same stroke volume, compared to constant outflow. This minimal additional energy associated with pulsatile ventricular ejection indicates the compliant properties of the receiving arterial tree.

An appreciable fraction of the energy in the pressure and flow pulses generated by the heart reaches the capillaries in pulsatile form. As seen in Fig. 4-44, pulsatility remains. This has been demonstrated experimentally by, e.g., Wiederhelm et al. (1964), in frog's mesentery; Intaglietta et al. (1970,1971), in cat omentum, Intaglietta and Zweifach, 1966; Zweifach (1974); Zweifach and Lipowsky (1977); and Smaje et al. (1980). It has been postulated that pulsations are necessary to attain optimal organ function. Steady perfusion could impair organ function (Wilkins et al., 1967; Jacobs et al., 1969; Arntzenius, 1976). Figure 4-44 illustrates direct recording of pressure obtained by Zweifach (1974). In the terminal arteriole, the pulse pressure is still large, about 15 mmHg, with a mean pressure of about 60 mmHg. Intaglietta et al. (1970) provided pulsatile velocity data. Mean velocities are in the centimeters-per-second (cm/s) range, as measured by electro-optical methods. The measurement of pressure and flow relationship and the assessment of human microvascular function, has been well addressed by Mayrovitz (1998), particularly on skin perfusion.

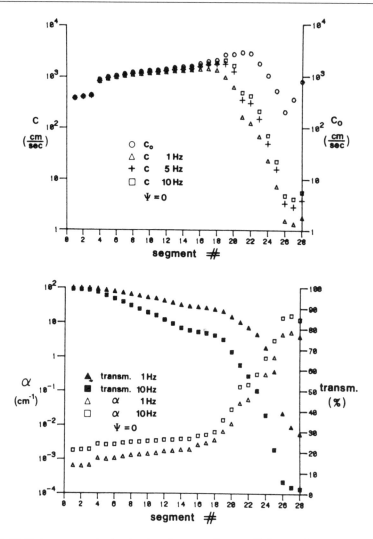

Fig. 4-46. Pulse wave velocity (top) and attenuation coefficient and percentage transmission at different frequencies shown, plotted as a function of transmission site from the ascending aorta to the index finger artery.

### 4.6.2. Pulse Transmission Characteristics in the Microcirculation

The steady flow concept assumed for the microcirculation is in accordance with the windkessel theory that peripheral vessels act as stiff tubes. This would protect the small vessels against sudden surges in flow and rapid changes in pressure.

With the advent of new technology, particularly the servo-controlled micropipet device for pressure measurement and electro-optical methods for velocity recording, studies of the pulse transmission in arterioles and capillaries became feasible. Although significantly damped, pressure and flow pulses generated by the heart persist into these vessels.

Caro et al. (1978) calculated a wave speed of 7.2 cm/s in the capillary with an exponential attenuation of 83%/cm. Estimated phase velocity from Intaglietta et al.'s (1971) data would give 7–10 cm/s, which is in general agreement. Caro et al. also gave an analytical expression for the propagation speed in the case of a sinusoidal pulse propagating through an elastic vessel, assuming blood is Newtonian:

$$c = \frac{1}{4}d \sqrt{[\omega/(\eta D)]} \qquad (4\text{-}58)$$

where $d$ is capillary diameter and $D$ is the distensibility. Since blood viscosity appears to decrease when measured in capillary tubes of decreasing diameter, blood, in fact, is non-Newtonian. This is known as the Fahraeus-Lindqvist effect (Li, 1987; Mayrovitz, 1998).

Li et al. (1980b) apparently were the first to provide analytical expressions to predict PWV and attenuation in the microcirculation. Linearized pulse transmission theory was utilized. Subsequently, the same group computed the pulse transmission from the LV to the human index finger vessel (Salotto et al., 1986; Fig. 4-45). Their computation was based on Westerhof's viscoelastic tube theory, with complex elastic modulus.

The results show wave velocity of a few centimeters per second and attenuation of about 30% at 1 Hz in large arterioles. With increasing frequencies, the attenuation becomes substantial, and pulse transmission is greatly reduced at 10 Hz (Fig. 4-46). This explains in part, why the observed pressure and flow waveforms, though pulsatile, are becoming more sinusoidal in the microcirculation.

## REFERENCES

Abel, F. L. Fourier analysis of left ventricular performance. Effect of impedance matching. *Circ. Res.* 28:119–135, 1971.

Alexander, R. S. Transformation of the arterial pulse wave between the aortic arch and the femoral artery. *Am. J. Physiol.* 158:287, 1949.

Alexander, R. S. The genesis of aortic standing wave. *Circ. Res.* 1:145–151, 1953.

Anliker, M., Histand, M. B., and Ogden, E. Dispersion and attenuation of small artificial pressure waves in the canine aorta. *Circ. Res.* 23:539–551, 1968.

Aperia, A. Haemodynamical studies. *Skand. Arch. Physiol.* 83 (Suppl. 1):1–230, 1940.

Arndt, J. O., Stegall, H. F., and Wicke, H. J. Mechanics of the aorta in vivo. *Circ. Res.* 28:693–704, 1971.

Arntzenius, A. C. Importance of pulsations. *Proc. CSDS Conf.,* Philadelphia, 1976.

Attinger, E. O., Anne, A., and McDonald, D. A. Use of Fourier series for the analysis of biological systems. *Biophys. J.* 6:291–304, 1966a.

Attinger, E. O., Sugawara, H., Nvarro, A., Ricetto, A., and Martin, R. Pressure-flow relations in dog arteries. *Circ. Res.* 19:230–246, 1966b.

Avolio, A. P., O'Rourke, M. F., Mang, K., Bason, P. T., and Gow, B. S. Comparative study of pulsatile arterial hemodynamics in rabbits and guinea pigs. *Am. J. Physiol.* 230:868–875, 1976.

Baan, J. *Transverse Impedance of Arteries: Animal Eexperiments Related to Wave Transmission Theory*. Ph. D. dissertation, University of Pennsylvania, Philadelphia, 1970.

Barnett, G. O., Maillos, A. J., and Shapiro, A. Relationship of aortic pressure and diameter in the dog. *J. Appl. Physiol.* 16:545, 1961.

Bergel, D. H. Dynamic elastic properties of the arterial wall. *J. Physiol.* 156:458–469, 1961.

Bergel, D. H. and Milnor, W. R. Pulmonary vascular impedance in the dog. *Circ. Res.* 16:401–415, 1965.

Bramwell, J. C. and A. V. Hill. The velocity of the pulse wave in man. *Proc. Roy. Soc. Lond. Biol.* 93:298–306, 1922.

Busse, R., Bauer, R. D., Schaben, A., Summa, Y., and Wettere, E. Improved method for the determination of the pulse transmission characteristics of arteries in vivo. *Circ. Res.* 44:630–636, 1979.

Caro, C. G., Bergel, D. H., and Seed, W. A. Forward and backward transmission of pressure waves in the pulmonary vascular bed of the dog. *Circ. Res.* 20:185–193, 1967.

Caro, C. G., Fitz-Gerald, J. M., and Schroter, R. C. Atheroma and arterial wall shear. *Proc. Roy. Soc. London* B177:109–159, 1971.

Caro, C. G. and McDonald, D. A. Relation of pulsatile pressure and flow in the pulmonary vascular bed. *J. Physiol.* 157:426–453, 1961.

Caro, C. G., Pedley, T. J., Schroter, R. C., and Seed, W. A. *Mechanics of the Circulation.* Oxford University Press, Oxford, 1978.

Clarke, T. N. S., Prys-Roberts, C., Biro, G., Foex, P., and Bennett, M. J. Aortic input impedance and left ventricular energetics in acute isovolumic anemia. *Cardiovasc. Res.* 12:49–55, 1978.

Cox, R. H. Blood flow and pressure propagation in the canine femoral artery. *J. Biomech.* 3:131–149, 1970.

Cox, R. H. Determination of the true phase velocity of arterial pressure waves in vivo. *Circ. Res.* 29:407–418, 1971.

Cox, R. H. Pressure dependence of the mechanical properties of arteries in vivo. *Am. J. Physiol.* 229:1371–1375, 1975.

Cox, R. H. and Pace, J. B. Pressure-flow relations in the vessels of the canine aortic arch. *Am. J. Physiol.* 228:1–10, 1975.

Dick, D. E., Kendrick, J. E., Matson, G. L., and Rideout, V. C. Measurement of nonlinearity in the arterial system of the dog by a new method. *Circ. Res.* 22:101, 1968.

Dow, P. and Hamilton, W. F. Experimental study of the velocity of the pulse wave propagated through the aorta. *Am. J. Physiol.* 125:60–65, 1939.

Dujardin, J.-P., Stone, D. N., Paul, L. T., and Pieper, H. P. Response of systemic arterial input impedance to volume expansion and hemorrhage. *Am. J. Physiol.* 238:H902–H908, 1980.

Evans, C. L. and Matsuoka, Y. Effect of various mechanical conditions on the gaseous metabolism and efficiency of the mammalian heart. *J. Physiol.* 49:378–405, 1915.

Fry, D. L., Griggs, D. M., Jr., and Greenfield, I. C., Jr. In vivo studies of pulsatile blood flow:The relationship of the pressure gradient to the blood velocity. In: Attinger, E. O., ed., *Pulsatile Blood Flow,* McGraw-Hill, New York, pp. 101–114, 1964.

Gabe, I. T., Gault, H. J., Ross, J., Jr., Mason, D. T., Mills, C. J., Shillingford, J. P., and Braunwaid, E. Measurement of instantaneous blood flow velocity and pressure in conscious man with a catheter-tip velocity probe. *Circulation* 40:603–614, 1964.

Gabe, I. T., Kamell, J., Porje, I. G,, and Rudewald, B. Measurement of input impedance and apparent phase velocity in the human aorta. *Acta Physiol. Scand.* 61:73–84, 1964.

Gessner, U. and Bergel, D. H. Methods of determining the distensibility of blood vessels. *IEEE Trans. Biomed. Eng.* BME-13:2–10, 1966.

Gosling, R. G., Newman, D. L., Bowden, N. L. R., and Twinn, K. W. Aortic configuration and pulse wave reflection. *Br. J. Radiol.* 44:850–853, 1971.

Grashey, H. Die Welienbewegung elastischer Rohren und der Arterienpuls des Merschen. Vogel Verlag, Leipzig, 1881.

Greenfield, J. C., Jr. and Fry, D. L. Relationship between instantaneous aortic flow and the pressure gradient. *Circ. Res.* 17:340–348, 1965.

Hagan, G. H. L. Uber die Bewegung des Wassers in engen cylindrischen Rohren. *Ann. Phys. Chem.* 46:423–444, 1839.

Hamilton, W. F. and Dow, P. Experimental study of the standing waves in the pulse propagated through the aorta. *Am. J. Physiol.* 125:48–59, 1939.

Hunt, W. A. Calculations of pulsatile flow across bifurcations in distensible tubes. *Biophys. J.* 9:993, 1969.

Intaglietta, M., Parvula, R. F., and Thompkins, W. R. Pressure measurements in the mammalian microvasculature. *Microvasc. Res.* 2:212–220, 1970.

Intaglietta, M., Richardson, D. R., and Thompkins, W. R. Blood pressure, flow, and elastic properties in microvessels of cat omentum. *Am. J. Physiol.* 221:922–928, 1971.

Intaglietta, M. and Zweifach, V. W. Indirect method for measurement of pressure in blood capillaries. *Circ. Res.* 19:199–205, 1966.

Jacobs, L. A., Klopp, E. H., Seamore, W., Topaz, S. R., and Gott, V. L. Improved organ functions during cardiac bypass with a roller pump modified to deliver pulsatile flow. *J. Thorac. Cardiovasc. Surg.* 58:703–712, 1969.

Kapal, E., Martini, F., and Wetterer, E. Uber die Zuverlassigkeit der bisherigen Bestimmungsart der Pulswellen geschwindigkeit. *Z. Biol.* 104:75–86, 1951.

Karamanoglu M., O'Rourke, M., Avolio, A. O., et al. Analysis of the relationship between central aortic and peripheral upper limb pressure waves in man. *Eur. Heart J.* 14:160–167, 1993.

Karreman, G. Some contributions to the mathematical biology of blood circulation: reflection of pressure waves in the arterial system. *Bull. Math. Biophys.* 14:327–350, 1952.

Krovetz, L. J., Jennings, R. B., Jr., and Goldbloom, S. D. Limitations of corrections of frequency dependent artifact in pressure recordings using harmonic analysis. *Circulation* 50:992–997, 1974.

Laszt, L. and Muller, A. Gleichzeitige Druckmessung in der Aorta abdominalis und ihren Hauptasten. *Helv. Physiol. Pharm. Acta* 10:259–272, 1952.

Laskey, W. K., Kussmaul, W. G., Martin, J. L., et al. Characteristics of vascular hydraulic load in patients with heart failure. *Circulation* 72:61–71, 1985.

Laskey W. K. and W. G. Kussmaul. Arterial wave reflections in heart failure. *Circ.* 75:711–722, 1987.

Latham, R. D., Westehof, N., and Sipkema, P. Regional wave travel and reflections along the human aorta: a study with six simultatneous micromanometric presures. *Circulation* 72:1257–1269, 1985.

Learoyd, B. M. and Taylor, M. G. Alterations with age in the viscoelastic properties of human arterial walls. *Circ. Res.* 18:278–292, 1966.

Lei, C. Q., Li, J. K.-J., Quick, C. Comparison of time domain and frequency domain assessments of arterial wave reflections. *Proc. 22nd. NE Bioeng. Conf.* 22:7–8, 1996.

Li, J. K.-J. *Mammalian Hemodynamics: Wave Transmission Characteristics and Similarity Analysis.* Ph. D. dissertation, University of Pennsylvania, Philadelphia, 1978.

Li, J. K.-J. Time domain resolution of forward and reflected waves in the aorta. *IEEE Trans. Biomed. Eng.* BME-33:783–785, 1986.

Li, J. K.-J. Pulse wave reflections at the aorto-iliac junction. *Angiology, J. Vasc. Dis.* 36:516–521, 1985.

Li, J. K.-J. Dominance of geometric aver elastic factors in pulse transmission through arterial branching. *Bull. Math. Biol.* 48:97–103, 1986b.

Li, J. K.-J. Increased arterial pulse wave reflections and pulsatile energy loss in acute hypertension. *Angiology, J. Vasc. Dis.* 40:730–735, 1989.

Li, J. K.-J. Cardiovascular diagnostic parameters derived from pressure and flow pulses. *Frontiers Eng. Healthcare* 4:186–189, 1982.

Li, J. K.-J. *Arterial System Dynamics.* New York University Press, New York, 1987.

Li, J. K.-J. New similarity principle for cardiac energetics. *Bull. Math. Biol.* 45:1005–1011, 1983.

Li, J. K.-J. *Comparative Cardiovascular Dynamics of Mammals.* CRC Press, New York, 1996.

Li, J. K.-J., Melbin, J., Campbell, K., and Noordergraaf, A. Evaluations of a three-point pressure method for the determination of arterial transmission characteristics. *J. Biomech.* 13:1023–1029, 1980a.

Li, J. K.-J., Melbin, J., and Noordergraaf, A. Pulse transmission to vascular beds. *Proc. 33rd ACEMB* 22:109, 1980b.

Li, J. K.-J., Melbin, J., and Noordergraaf, A. Optimality of pulse transmission at vascular branching junctions. *Cardiovasc. Syst. Dynamics* 6:228–230, 1984a.

Li, J. K.-J., Melbin, J., and Noordergraaf, A. Directional disparity of pulse wave reflections in dog arteries. *Am. J. Physiol.* 247:495–499, 1984b.

Li, J. K.-J., Melbin, J., Riffle, R. A., and Noordergraaf, A. Pulse wave propagation. *Circ. Res.* 49:442–452, 1981.

Ling, S. C., Atabek, H. B., Letzing, W. G., and Patel, D. J. Nonlinear analysis of aortic flow in living dogs. *Circ. Res.* 33:198–212, 1973.

Luchsinger, P. C., Snell, R. E., Patel, D. J., and Fry, D. L. Instantaneous pressure distribution among the human aorta. *Circ. Res.* 15:503–510, 1964.

McDonald, D. A. and Taylor, M. G. Hydrodynamics of the arterial circulation. *Progr. Biophys. Biophys. Chem.* 9:105,107–173, 1959.

McDonald, D. A. *Blood Flow in Arteries.* Arnold, London, 1960.

McDonald, D. A. *Blood Flow in Arteries.* Arnold, London, 1974.

McDonald, D. A. Regional pulse-wave velocity in the arterial tree. *J. Appl. Physiol.* 24:73–78, 1968.

McDonald, D. A., and Gessner, U. Wave attenuation in viscoelastic arteries. In: *Copley, A. L., ed., Hemorheology,* Pergamon Press, Oxford, pp. 113-125, 1968.

Malindzak, G. S. Fourier analysis of cardiovascular events. *Math. Biosci.* 7:273, 1970.

Maxwell, J. A. and Anliker, M. The dissiparrions and dispersion of small waves in arteries and veins with viscoelastic wall properties. *Biophys. J.* 8:920–950, 1968.

Mayrovitz, H. N. Assessment of human microvascular function. In: Drzewieki, G. and Li, J. K.-J., eds., *Analysis and Assessment of Cardiovascular Function,* Springer-Verlag, New York, pp. 248–273, 1998.

Mills, C. J., Gabe, I. T., Gault, J. H., Mason, D. T., Ross, J., Braunwald, E., and Shillingford, J. P. Pressure-flow relationships and vascular impedance in man. *Cardiovasc. Res.* 4:405–417, 1970.

Milnor, W. R. Arterial impedance as ventricular afterload. *Circ. Res.* 36:565–570, 1975.

Milnor, W. R. and Bertram, C. D. Relation between arterial viscoelasticity and wave propagation in the canine femoral artery in vivo. *Circ. Res.* 43:870–879, 1978.

Milnor, W. R. and Nichols, W. W. New method of measuring propagation coefficients and characteristic impedance in blood vessels. *Circ. Res.* 36:631–639, 1975.

Murgo, J. P., Westerhof, N., Giolma, J. P., and Altobelli, S. A. Aortic input impedance in normal man:relationship to pressure waveforms. Circu*lation* 62:105–116, 1980.

Murgo, J. P., Westerhof, N., Giolma, J. P., and Altobelli, S. A. Manipulation of ascending aortic pressure and flow wave reflections with the Valsalva maneuver: relationship to input impedance. *Circulation* 63:122–132, 1981.

Newman, D. L., Batten, J. R., and Bowden, N. L. R. Partial standing wave formations above an abdominal aortic stenosis. *Cardiovasc. Res.* 11:160, 1977.

Newman, D. L. and Bowden, N. L. R. Effect of reflection from an unmatching junction of the abdominal aortic impedance. *Cardiovasc. Res.* 7:827, 1973.

Newman, D. L., Greenwald, S. E., and N. L. R. Bowden. In vivo study of the total occlusion method for the analysis of forward and backward pressure waves. *Cardiovasc. Res.* 13:595–600, 1979.

Nichols, W. W., Conti, C. R., Walker, W. E., and Milnor, W. R. Input impedance of the systematic circulation in man. *Circ. Res.* 40:451–458, 1977.

Nichols, W. W. and McDonald, D. A. Wave velocity in the proximal aorta. *Med. Biol. Eng.* 10:327–335, 1972.

Noble, M. I. M., Gabe, I. T., and Guz, A. Blood pressure and flow in the ascending of conscious dogs. *Cardiovasc. Res.* 1:9–0, 1967.

Noordergraaf, A. *Circulatory System Dynamics.* Academic, New York, 1978.

O'Rourke, M. F. Pressure and flow waves in systemic arteries and the anatomical design of the arterial system. *J. Appl. Physiol.* 23:139–149, 1967.

O'Rourke, M. F. Impact pressure, lateral pressure, and impedance in the proximal aorta and pulmonary artery. *J. Appl. Physiol.* 25:533–541, 1968.

O'Rourke, M. F. and Taylor, M. G. Vascular impedance of the femoral bed. *Circ. Res.* 18:126–139, 1966.

O'Rourke, M. F. and Taylor, M. G. Input impedance of the systemic circulation. *Circ. Res.* 20:365–380, 1967.

Patel, D. J., DeFreitas, F. M., and Fry, D. L. Hydraulic input impedance to aorta and pulmonary artery in dogs. *J. Appl. Physiol.* 18:134–140, 1963.

Patel, D. J., Greenfield, J. C., Jr., Austen, W. G., Morrow, A. G., and Fry, D. L. Pressure–flow relationships in the ascending aorta and femoral artery of man. *J. Appl. Physiol.* 20:459–463, 1965.

Peluso, F., Topham, W. S. and Noordergraaf, A. Response of systemic input impedance to exercise and graded aortic constriction. In: Baan, J., Noordergraaf, A., and Raines, J., eds., *Cardiovascular System Dynamics,* MIT Press, Cambridge, pp. 432–440, 1978.

Peterson, L. H. and Gerst, P. H. Significance of reflected waves within the arterial system. *Fed. Proc.* 15:144, 1956.

Poiseuliie, J. L. M. Recherches experimentales sur le mouvement des liquides dan les tubes de tres petit diameters. *C. R. Acad. Sci.* 12:112, 1841.

Porje, I. G. Studies of the arterial pulse wave, particularly in the aorta. *Acta. Physiol. Scand.* 42Suppl:1–68, 1946.

Porje, I. G. Energy design of the human circulatory system. *Cardiology* 51:293–306, 1967.

Randall, J. E. and Stacy, R. W. Mechanical impedance of the dog's hind leg to pulsatile blood flow. *Am. J. Physiol.* 187:94–98, 1956.

Remington, J. W. Physiology of the aorta and major arteries. In: *Handbook of Physiology,* vol. 2, American Physiologial Society, Washington, DC, 1963.

Remington, J. W. and Wood, E. H. Formations of peripheral pulse contour in man. *J. Appl. Physiol.* 9:433, 1956.

Reuben, S. R., Swadling, J. P., Gersh, B. J., and Lee, G. de J. Impedance and transmission properties of the pulmonary arterial system. *Cardiovasc. Res.* 5:1–9, 1971.

Rockwell, R. L., Anliker, M., and Ogden, E. Shock waves and other nonlinear phenomena of wave propagation in blood vessels. *Proc. IOMBE* 6:4, 1969.

Rodbard, S., Williams, F., and Williams, C. Spherical dynamics of the heart. *Am. Heart J.* 57:348–360, 1959.

Safar, M. E., Simon, A. C., and Levenson, J. A. Structural changes of large arteries in sustained essential hypertension. *Hypertension* 6(SIII):117–121, 1984.

Salotto, A., Muscarella, L. F., Melbin, J., Li, J. K-J., and Noordergraaf, A. Pressure pulse transmission into vascular beds. *Microvasc. Res.* 32:152–163, 1986.

Sarpkaya, T. Reflections and transmissions of pulse waves in distensible bifurcating vessels. *Dig. 7th ICMBE*, 1967.

Shi, W.-M. and Li, J. K.-J. Time and frequency domain determination of the characteristic impedance of the aorta. *Proc. 11th NE Bioeng. Conf.* 11:1–2, 1985.

Simon, A. C., and Levenson, J. Use of arterial compliance for evaluation of hypertenion. *Am. J. Hypertens.* 3:97–105, 1990.

Smaje, L. H., Fraser, P. A., and Clough, G. Distensibility of single capillaries and venules in the cat mesentery. *Microvasc. Res.* 20:358–370, 1980.

Solmyo, A. V. and Solmyo, A. P. Electrocmechanical and pharmaco-mechanical couling in cascular smooth muscle. *J. Pharmacol. Exp. Therp.* 159:129–145, 1968.

Spencer, M. P. and Denison, A. B. The aortic flow pulse as related to differential pressure. *Circ. Res.* 4:476–484, 1956.

Spengler, L. Symbolae et theoriam de sanguinis arteriosi fluimine. Dissertation, University of Marburg, Marburg, 1843.

Sperling, W., Bauer, R. D., Busse, R., Komer, H., and Pasch, Th. Resolution of arterial pulses into forward and backward waves as an approach to the determination of the characteristic impedance. *Pflugers Arch.* 355:217, 1975.

Taylor, M. G. An approach to the analysis of the arterial pulse wave. 1. Oscillations in an attenuating line. *Phys. Med. Biol.* 1:258–269, 1957.

Taylor, M. G. Use of random excitation and spectral analysis in the study of frequency-dependent parameters of the cardiovascular system. *Circ. Res.* 18:585–595, 1966.

Van den Bos, G. C., Westerhof, N., Eizinga, G., and Sipkema, P. Reflection in the systemic arterial system:effects of aortic and carotid occlusion. *Cardiovasc. Res.* 10:565–573, 1976.

Van den Bos, G. C., Westerhof, N., and Randall, O. S. Pulse wave reflection: can it explain the differenes between systematic and pulmonary pressure and flow waves? *Circ. Res.* 51:470–485, 1982.

Von Kries, J. *Studien zur Pulslehre.* Akad. Verlag, Freiberg, 1892.

Wells S. M., Langeille, B. L., and Adamson, S. L. In vivo and in vitro mechanical properties of the sheep in thoracic aorta in the perinatal period and adulthood. *Am. J. Physiol.* 274:H1749–H1760, 1998.

Westerhof, N., Bosman, F., DeVries, C. J., and Noordergraaf, A. Analog studies of the human systemic arterial tree. *J. Biomech.* 2:121–143, 1969.

Westerhof, N., Eizinga, G., and Van den Bos, G. C. Influence of central and peripheral changes on the hydraulic input impedance of the systemic arterial tree. *Med. Biol. Eng.* 11:710–723, 1973.

Westerhof, N., Sipkema, P., Van Den Bos, G. C., and Eizinga, G. Forward and backward waves in the arterial system. *Cardiovasc. Res.* 6:648–656, 1972.

Wetterer, E. and Kenner, T. *Grundlagen der Dynamik des Arterienpulses.* Springer-Verlag, Berlin, 1968.

Wetterer, E., Bauer, R. and Busse, R. New ways of determining the propagation coefficient and the viscoelastic behavior of arteries in situ. In: Bauer, R. D. and Busse, R., eds., *The Arterial System,* Springer-Verlag, Berlin, pp. 35–47, 1978.

Wiederhelm, C. A., Woodbury, J. W., Kirk, S., and Rushmer, R. F. Pulsatile pressure in the microcirculation of the frog's mesentery. *Am. J. Physiol.* 207:173–176, 1964.

Wiggers, C. J. *Pressure Pulses in the Cardiovascular System.* Longmans, London, 1928.

Wilkins, H., Regdson, W., and Hoffmeister, F. S. The physiological importance of pulsatile blood flow. *New Engl. J. Med.* 267:443–445, 1967.

Womersley, J. R. Oscillatory flow in arteries: the reflections of the pulse wave at junctions and rigid inserts in the arterial system. *Phys. Med. Biol.* 2:313–323, 1958.

Zamir, M. Local geometry of arterial branching. *Bull. Math. Biol.* 44:597–607, 1982.

Zweifach, B. W. Quantitative studies of microcirculatory structure and functions. *Circ. Res.* 34:858–866, 1974.

Zweifach, B. W. and Lipowsky, H. H. Quantitative studies of microcirculatory structure and function. III. Microcirculatory hemodynamics of cat mesentery and rabbit omentum. *Circ. Res.* 41:380, 1977.

# 5 Hemodynamic Measurements and Clinical Monitoring

## 5.1. Invasive Blood Pressure Measurements

The fluid-filled catheter-manometer system (CMS) continues to be the most common approach to invasive monitoring of pulsatile blood pressure (BP) waveforms in cardiac chambers and major vessels of the circulation. This is because of the long, well-established, and improved catheterization techniques, in combination with angiographic imaging modalities in the clinical catheterization laboratories. The catheter system has the added advantage of the ease of injecting radiopaque dyes for visualization of the vasculature, as well as administering therapeutical drugs. Balloon catheter for angioplasty applications and local intravascular drug delivery have also become popular. More recent multi-functional catheters include thermodilution, as well as the addition of electrodes for either atrial or ventricular pacing capabilities. These technological advances have promoted the popularity of interventional cardiology.

The catheter was originally introduced in man by Forssmann (1929) in a peripheral artery. Cournand and Range (1941) advanced the catheter from a peripheral vessel to the heart, and established an early catherization method for measurement of right heart pressure. Accuracy of BP measurements by invasive means, with the combination of catheter and manometer, has since been analyzed by several investigators (e.g., Hansen, 1949; Fry et al., 1957; Latimer, 1968; Li et al., 1976; Li and Noordergraaf, 1977). Additional evaluation has also been performed for double-lumen catheters connected to pressure transducers or manometers.

The catheter has the flexibility and maneuverability that allows accessibility to different parts of the circulation. There are instances in which a combination of a hypodermic needle and a pressure transducer suffices, particularly when the blood vessel is superficial or under intraoperative conditions. Brachial or femoral arteries are common superficial sites for pressure measurements with needle–transducers. Left ventricular (LV) chamber pressure measurement with apex insertion of a needle is also common under open-chest conditions.

From: *Arterial Circulation: Physical Principles and Clinical Applications*
By: J. K-J. Li © Humana Press Inc., Totowa, NJ

In fluid-filled BP measurement systems, the needle–manometer combination possesses a superior frequency response, compared to a catheter-manometer combination, because of the stiffness of the needle. However, care still must be taken in the choice of needle size and pressure transducer, so that adequate frequency response may be obtained to reproduce cardiac or arterial blood pressure waveforms faithfully.

## 5.1.1. The Needle–Manometer System (NMS)

The representation of the needle–manometer system (NMS) has been in two general forms: mechanical and electrical. The simplest representation is an undamped spring–mass system of natural frequency:

$$f_n = \frac{1}{2\pi} \sqrt{\frac{\pi r^2}{\rho l} \times \frac{dp}{dV}}$$

(5-1)

where $r$ is the internal lumen radius of the needle, $l$ is the length of the needle, and $\rho$ is the fluid density. Typically the needle and pressure transducer dome are filled with saline, which provides the required fluid coupling that is necessary when the needle is inserted into an artery. Heparine is often added to prevent clotting. Blood pressure pulsation is transmitted via fluid coupling, resulting in the movement of the pressure transducer diaphragm. The greater the amount of fluid, the greater the fluid movement or inertia. Thus, the inertia is represented by

$$L = \frac{\rho l}{\pi r^2}$$

(5-2)

The compliance of the manometer (volume displacement per unit distending pressure in units of mL/mmHg, or mL/10 cm $H_2O$) is determined by the stainless steel diaphragm within the fluid-filled transducer dome. Compliance is the inverse of stiffness:

$$C = \frac{dV}{dp} = \frac{1}{dp/dV} = \frac{1}{stiffness}$$

(5-3)

Thus, a more compliant pressure transducer means that volume displacement ($dV$) of its diaphragm is greater when subjected to the same amount of applied pressure ($dp$). The consequence of this, in the accuracy of BP recording is explained below. The compliance of the needle (stainless steel with high Young's modulus of elasticity and therefore, very stiff) is negligible. Equation 5-1 can be rewritten as

$$f_n = \frac{1}{2\pi} \sqrt{\frac{1}{LC}}$$

(5-4)

This representation is shown in Fig. 5-1 (A). When the needle is small, the Poiseuille resistance, $R$, becomes important in the determination of the frequency response. An improved second-order representation is shown in Fig. 5-1 (B), when the inertia becomes important.

Because the arterial pressure is periodic, and can be written as the sum of the mean pressure, $\overline{p}$ and the sum of a number of sine waves of fundamental frequency, $f$ (heart rate/s), and harmonics, $nf$ ($n = 1,2, \ldots, N$), then the arterial or cardiac pressure, waveform can be represented in a Fourier series, as discussed in the previous chapter:

$$p(t) = \overline{p} + \sum_{n=1}^{N} p_n \sin(n\omega t + \phi_n) \qquad (5\text{-}5)$$

which, when substituted into the second order differential equation describing the fluid motion, results in the amplitude ratio for the nth harmonic:

$$\frac{P_{mn}}{P_{on}} = \sqrt{\frac{1}{1 - (n\omega)^2 LC + (n\omega RC)^2}} \qquad (5\text{-}6)$$

and the corresponding phase angle is

$$\phi_n = \tan^{-1} \frac{n\omega RC}{1 - n\omega LC} \qquad (5\text{-}7)$$

$$\omega = 2\pi f \qquad (5\text{-}8)$$

where $P_{mn}$ = measured pressure for the nth harmonic and $P_{on}$ = actual pressure of the nth harmonic component. For a distortion-free NMS, or one with a flat frequency response, it is necessary that the amplitude ratio $P_{mn}/P_{on}$ be unity, or there is no difference between the pressure measured by the transducer and the actual blood pressure. Under this condition, the phase angle $\phi_n = 0$, i.e., there is no phase shift between measured pressure and actual pressure. Equations 5-6 and 5-7 represent the second-order approximation of the frequency response of the NMS. The corresponding electrical analogy, or the series combination of RLC, is shown in Fig. 5-1(B).

For the pressure measurement system to record the arterial blood pressure waveform faithfully, it must have sufficient dynamic frequency response. For the needle–manometer, it often results in changing the needle size or length of the needle, when an additional pressure transducer of different compliance specifications is unavailable. From the above expressions, it can be seen that increasing the needle radius or reducing its length can significantly improve the frequency response. The frequency responses of the various combinations of needle–pressure transducer systems are given by Li et al. (1976). Needle-manometer systems usually have sharper resonant peaks than their catheter–manometer counterparts.

**A**

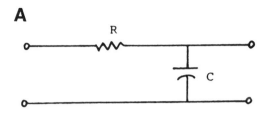

**B**

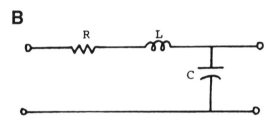

Fig 5-1. **(A)** The NMS represented by a lumped RC circuit (spring-dashpot). $R$ = resistance, $C$ = compliance of the manometer. **(B)** NMS represented by a lumped RLC circuit. $L$ = inertia of fluid, $C$ = compliance of the manometer, and $R$ = Poiseuille resistance.

The propagation constant measurements calculated from the three-point pressure method shown in Chapter 4 actually utilized three identical needle-manometer systems, each of which consists of a 5-cm 22-gage needle in combination with a P23Gb pressure transducer mounted on a stereotaxic manifold. NMS are easier to match than CMS, because of the shorter length and stiffness of the needle. Differential pressures and pressure gradients can be more accurately measured with matched needle–pressure trans-ducer combinations (Li and Noordergraaf, 1977; Li et al.,1978). Figure 5-2 illustrates the designs of the L-needles, which have been used to obtain pressure gradients in the femoral artery, the carotid artery, and the main pulmonary trunk.

### 5.1.2. CATHETER-MANOMETER SYSTEMS (CMS)

The use of catheters in man derives from Forssmann's (1929) idea on how to inject fluid and drugs into a vein close to the heart of a critically ill patient. The catheter was subsequently used for the withdrawal of blood samples (Cournand and Ranges, 1941), as well as for injection of solutions. Remote sensing of BP by means of a catheter became popular in both physiological research and clinical investigation. It affords continuous recording of blood pressure waveforms at virtually any site in the cardio-vascular system, outside the microvasculature.

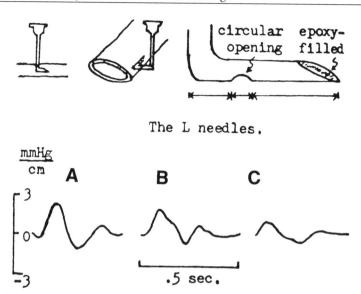

Fig. 5-2. Pressure gradients in the (**A**) femoral artery, (**B**) carotid artery, and (**C**) main pulmonary trunk, measured with specially designed L-needles, in combination with pressure transducers.

For a catheter-manometer system, frequently an underdamped system, compliance as well as geometric, factors such as length and radius of the catheter are important. Figure 5-3 provides a lumped approximation of the system.

Experimental evaluations of manometric system response usually employ either a sinusoidal pressure generator (Stegall et al., 1968) or the "pop-test." In this latter test, a step increase in pressure is applied against the catheter-transducer system, and the balloon, which is connected to the same chamber as the catheter, is inflated. The balloon is then rapidly "popped" with a sharp needle. The pressure in the chamber thus falls to atmospheric pressure, completing the step decrease in pressure. If the CMS had a perfect dynamic response, then its response would follow exactly the step decline in pressure. However, clinically and experimentally used catheter–transducer combinations are usually underdamped, resulting in oscillations.

The damped natural resonance frequency, $f_d$, is obtained as the inverse of the period of oscillation:

$$f_d = 1/T \tag{5-9}$$

where $T$ is the period of oscillation. This can be obtained from the interval of the peak-to-peak oscillation.

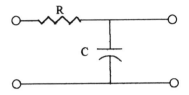

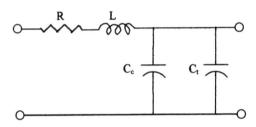

Fig. 5-3. Lumped model representation of the CMS. (Top) Lumped RC circuit. $R =$ Poiseuille resistance of the fluid in the catheter, $C =$ compliance combination of the catheter and the manometer $(C_c + C_t)$. (Bottom) Lumped series RLC circuit, with $L =$ inertia of fluid, $C_c =$ compliance of the catheter, and $C_t =$ compliance of the transducer.

The exponential damping, $\alpha_e$ is determined from the peak amplitudes, $A_1$ and $A_2$,

$$A_1/A_2 = e^{-\alpha_e t} \tag{5-10}$$

or, in terms of amplitude ratio, $A_p$,

$$A_p = \ln(A_2/A_1) \tag{5-11}$$

The relative damping factor, $\alpha_d$, is obtained from the following expression:

$$\alpha_d = \frac{A_p}{\sqrt{4\pi^2 + A_p^2}} \tag{5-12}$$

In general, experimentally and clinically used CMS exhibit under-damped responses in which the damping factors are typically 0.2–0.3. A simple rule of thumb is to estimate the useful frequency range by multiplying the resonant frequency by the damping factor. For example, if the resonant frequency is 40 Hz and the damping factor is 0.25, then the "flat frequency" response is to $40 \times 0.25$, or 10 Hz. The flat frequency response refers to an amplitude ratio (Eq. 5-6) within ±5% of unity, or 1. In other words, the measured pressure is within ±5% of the actual pressure. Thus,

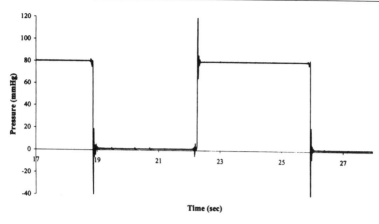

Fig. 5-4. Dynamic testing of blood pressure measurement systems with either a positive or a negative step. Overshoot and oscillations are seen.

higher resonant frequencies and greater damping factors (up to critical damping) offer better dynamic frequency response.

The step response, or pop-test, has advantages of simplicity and rapid tracking of system response. This method is shown in Fig. 5-4. One can apply either a positive step (step increment in pressure) or a negative step (step decrement in pressure). An ideal BP measurement system follows the step exactly, with no overshoot or undershoot, and no time delay. In practice, however, overshoot and oscillations are common. Figure 5-5 illustrates the underdamped response of a fluid-filled CMS.

The dynamic frequency response, in terms of relative amplitude ratio vs frequency for the step response of Fig. 5-5, is shown in Fig. 5-6. The single resonance peak occurs as the underdamped CMS was approximated by the second-order system. For details on the response of second order systems, one should consult standard textbooks (e.g., Hyatt and Kemmerly, 1978; Nilsson, 1983). In general, linearity, hysteresis, and dynamic system response are necessary considerations in fluid-filled BP measurement systems. Linearity refers to the output response vs input applied pressure. This is not generally a problem, because most combinations have static calibrations that are linear to within ±1%, or better, over the range of 0–200 mmHg. Hysteresis refers to the differences in outputs with increasing and decreasing BP within the BP range of interest. This is also typically small. Thus, dynamic frequency response is of major importance.

Blood pressure waveforms that are closer to sinusoidal waveforms require fewer harmonic components to resynthesize the original waveform, and thus place less stringent demand on the frequency response. For instance, the femoral artery can be recorded with a lower dynamic fre-

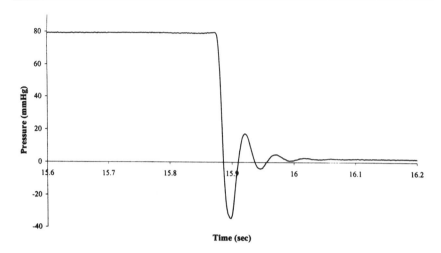

Fig. 5-5. The pop-test (step response) for the dynamic testing of transducer system performance, $f = {}^1/_T$ = resonant frequency. The catheter–transducer system is seen to be an underdamped system.

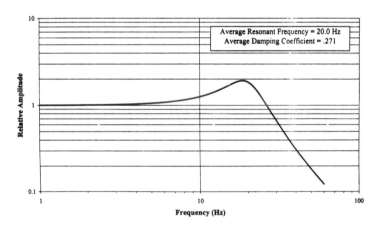

Fig. 5-6. Dynamic frequency response shown as the relative amplitude ratio vs frequency. The resonance frequency in this example is 20 Hz.

quency response than either central aortic pressure (AoP) or LVP (Li and Matonick, 1998). This is because the femoral AP is generally smoother, with rounded incisura. BP waveforms that are closer to rectangular waveform require much higher frequency response, to resynthesize the waveforms accurately. This is because rectangular and square waves contain an infinite number of sinusoidal or cosinusoidal components. Normal LVP, for instance, contains much higher frequency components than the femoral

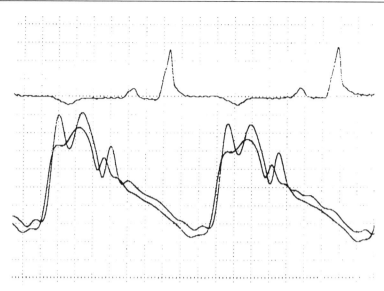

Fig. 5-7. Aortic blood pressure waveform measured with an underdamped CMS and a high-fidelity catheter-tip pressure transducer. Overshoot and oscillations are clearly seen.

AP. The first derivatives of pressure, such as LV dp/dt, also requires higher-frequency response for accurate recording.

When the blood pressure waveform is recorded with a low resonant frequency and low damping ratio, fluid-filled BP measurement system, erroneous phase shifts and large oscillations can be observed. Figure 5-7 illustrates this point, with the aortic pressure waveform measured simultaneously by a high-fidelity catheter-tip pressure transducer and a low-fidelity fluid-filled CMS. The two waveforms are calibrated and superimposed. Overestimation of systolic pressure and underestimation of diastolic pressure can be observed. In addition, end-systolic pressure at aortic valve closure, systolic, diastolic, and ejection periods cannot be accurately determined. This is also seen in the pressure measured a few cm distal (Fig. 5-8). The differences are clearly visible when the tracings are separated (Fig. 5-8).

Li et al. (1976) have analyzed the system response by representing the catheter with distributed properties, utilizing either $\Gamma$- (inverted-L) or $\pi$-network configurations shown in Figs. 5-9 and 5-10. Sets of equations that describe the fluid flow through an elastic tube were introduced. Various combinations of stiff and compliant catheters and manometers were studied. It was found that a combination of a stiff catheter and a low-volume displacement (stiff diaphragm) transducer provides the best frequency response (Fig. 5-11). Multiple resonance frequencies are observed when a

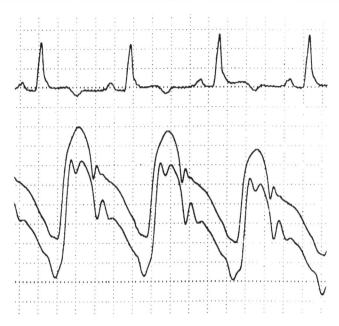

Fig. 5-8. Aortic blood pressure waveform measured with a catheter-tip pressure transducer system (upper) and a fluid-filled BP measurement system (lower). Tracings are shifted to clarify differences. Overshoots and pronounced oscillations can be seen in the lower tracing.

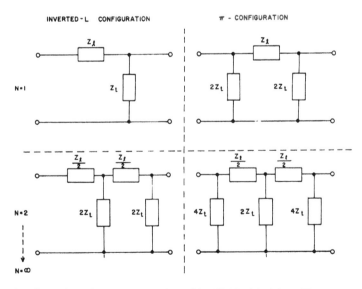

Fig. 5-9. Configuration of the representation of the CMS with either a $\Gamma$- or a $\pi$-network. Adapted with permission from Li et al. (1976).

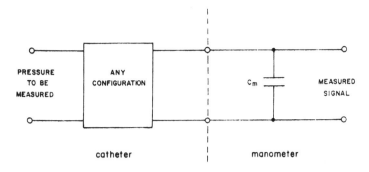

Fig. 5-10. Schematic illustration of any of the configurations of catheter in Fig. 5-9 in combination with a manometer with compliance $Cm$. Adapted with permission from Li et al. (1976).

catheter with large compliance, i.e., a very compliant catheter, is used in combination with a manometer. Methods used to improve damping are not worthwhile when applied to a system already possessing very poor frequency response. Therefore, the use of sophisticated digital or analog compensation techniques (Falsetti et al., 1974; Melbin and Spohr, 1969) should be restricted to cases in which only small corrections are required to extend the useful frequency response, and to cases in which multiple resonances do not occur at low frequencies.

Li and Noordergraaf (1977) have analyzed responses of differential manometer systems. For these systems, the individual frequency response, as well as static and dynamic imbalances, are important factors to be considered. Catheter-tip pressure transducers offer superior frequency response, sufficient even for cardiac sound recording. However, they suffer from fragility, temperature-sensitivity, and the need to be calibrated against known manometric systems. The efficacy of catheterization in the diagnostic setting has been discussed by Li and Kostis (1984).

## 5.2. Noninvasive Blood Pressure Measurements

### 5.2.1. Auscultatory Measurement of Blood Pressure

The most popular form of noninvasive BP measurement in the clinical setting remains that of the Korotkoff auscultatory method, which, however, lacks accuracy when compared to invasive catheter technique. Some 5–10 mmHg error is commonly found. Nevertheless, this technique is simple to employ, very convenient, and has high repeatability. It allows both systolic and diastolic pressures to be determined. Subsequently, the pulse pressure (PP) is obtained by subtraction of the two. We shall examine this method in more detail.

The Korotkoff sound method employs an occlusive cuff and a stethoscope. All occlusive cuff methods apply known air pressure to the upper

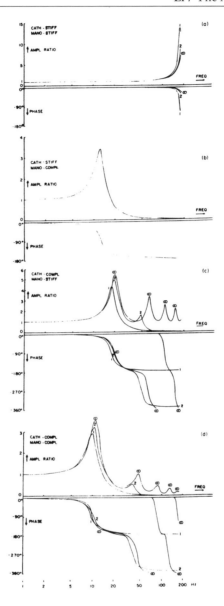

Fig. 5-11. Frequency responses of the various combinations of stiff and compliant catheters with stiff and compliant manometers (pressure transducers). Adapted with permission from Li et al. (1976).

arm, although other limbs, or the tail in animals, have been used. The method was first conceived by Riva-Rocci (1896). Korotkoff (1905) first demonstrated the modern-day auscultatory method, and suggested that

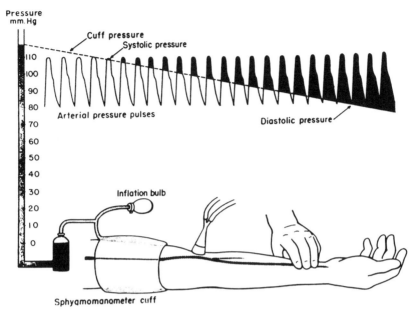

Fig. 5-12. Illustration of the auscultatory method for recording blood pressure. Adapted with permission from Rushmer (1972).

arterial collapse and opening was the reason for the occurrence of the vascular sounds.

The modern auscultatory method is illustrated in Fig. 5-12. The cuff is inflated to a pressure exceeding the expected systolic arterial pressure ($P_s$). During the inflation of the cuff, with cuff pressure exceeding that of the systolic pressure, the segment of the artery under the cuff is forced to collapse, either partially or completely. The cuff is then allowed to deflate slowly at a few mmHg/s, through a needle valve which allows air to escape, hence dropping the cuff pressure. During deflation, the initial arterial lumen opening that is detected is the systolic pressure. The first vascular sounds that emerge are generally referred to as phase I, define $P_s$. When either the vascular sounds become muffled (phase IV) or disappear completely (phase V), the diastolic pressure ($P_d$) is obtained. This technique has an estimated accuracy of 5–10 mmHg. There remains debate as to whether phase IV or V is a better indicator of diastolic pressure (Levine, 1981). Figure 5-13 illustrates the Korotkoff vascular sounds recorded in a brachial artery. When vascular reactivity is altered with handgrip, the spectral content is shifted, so that the Korotkoff sound intensity is increased, together with a higher observed BP (Rabbany et al., 1993; Matonick and Li, 1999). This is illustrated in Fig. 5-14.

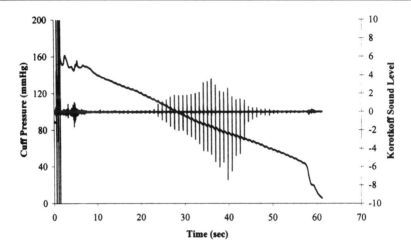

Fig. 5-13. Korotkoff vascular sounds recorded in a brachial artery.

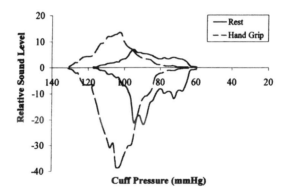

Fig. 5-14. Korotkoff sound cuff method when the vasoactivity is altered by fist-clinching. Provided by J. Matonick.

The width and length of the cuff are important considerations in the application of the auscultatory method (Karvonen et al., 1964; Simpson et al., 1965; Geddes and Whistler, 1978). A width-to-circumference ratio of 0.4 has been suggested (Kirkendall et al., 1981). There is an optimum width of the cuff: Narrower than optimum cuffs tend to impose an arterial stress below that of cuff pressure, and can result in an overestimation of BP; a cuff wider than optimum provides accurate recording only at the center of the cuff, and can cause error in detection, as stress declines away from the center, giving a lower estimation of pressure. For this, and other reasons, there are differences in the current design of adult and pediatric BP cuffs.

### 5.2.2. Oscillometric Method

Alternative to the use of the stethoscope is the oscillometric method. Over a century ago, Marey (1885) found that cuff pressure oscillated over a considerable range of mean cuff pressures. He suggested that the oscillation is maximal when the arterial wall is not stressed circumferentially. Removal of this circumferential stress, as seen in Subheading 5.2.5., provides a basis for noninvasive tonometry. In this "vascular unloading," as Marey termed it, the tension within the wall of the artery under such circumstance is zero, when the transmural pressure is zero. Such vascular unloading is fundamental to the occlusive cuff methods of BP determination.

This maximal oscillation was found to correspond to mean arterial pressure as observed in animal experiments (Posey et al., 1969) and in humans (Ramsey, 1979). The oscillometric method continued to gain popularity; although this technique is rather accurate for systolic and mean blood pressure detection, its accuracy is much less so for diastolic pressure measurement (Geddes et al., 1982).

Geddes (1984) has provided a detailed analysis and comparison of the cuff technique and oscillometry. Figure 5-15 shows the corresponding appearance and disappearance of the Korotkoff sounds and the oscillations in cuff pressure. Maximum oscillation in cuff pressure corresponds to mean blood pressure as shown. Thus, in addition to systolic and diastolic pressures, mean blood pressure can be obtained. The radial pulse distal to brachial artery measurement site is also shown.

### 5.2.3. Ultrsound Method

Arzbaecher and Novotney (1973) managed to synthesize arterial pressure waveform from the cuff, together with the appearance time of the Korotkoff sounds (Rodbard et al., 1957). On the other hand, the ultrasound Doppler method (e.g., Stegall et al., 1968) records BP waveform by detecting Doppler signals received as the motion of the blood vessel varies under different states of occlusion.

### 5.2.4. Automated Blood Pressure Measurements

Automated blood pressure measurement currently utilizes a microphone to sense the Korotkoff sounds or by oscillometric method (e.g., Mauer and Noordergraaff, 1976; Ramsey, 1983; Geddes and Baker, 1989; Ramsey, 1991). The microphone, which substitutes for the stethoscope, is normally placed over the brachial artery. Systolic blood pressure indicated by the phase I sound is detected in the 18–26 Hz range with a band-pass filter. Diastolic pressure in the phase IV sound is detected in the 40–60 Hz range. The use of microphone can provide an objective measure, irrespective of differences in hearing acuity, which varies among individuals. The hearing

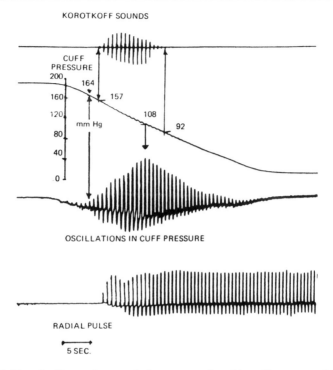

Fig. 5-15. Korotkoff sounds recorded concurrently with cuff pressure. Maximum oscillation in cuff pressure corresponds to mean blood pressure as shown. Radial arterial pulse distal to the brachial artery measurement site is also shown. Adapted with permission from Geddes (1984).

acuity plays an important role in differentiating the muffled vascular sounds occurring during the diastolic period. Automated BP recording has the advantage of providing continuous, noninvasive recording which has been in wide use in the ambulatory monitoring of BP.

Drzewiecki (1985) offered a theory to the origin of the Korotkoff sounds. The origins of Korotkoff sounds have been a controversial subject of research. Their origins are pressure-related, rather than flow-related (Drzewieki et al., 1987,1989).

### 5.2.5. Noninvasive Blood Pressure Monitoring and Arterial Tonometer

There are several methods for noninvasive recording of BP waveforms. Some of these, with some accuracy in registering superficial arterial pressure waveforms, date back to Marey's (1885) time. Those that have continued to the present included the volume pulse method, the pressure pulse method, and the cantilever and optical deflection methods.

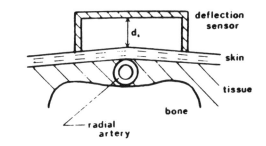

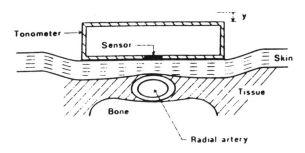

Fig. 5-16. Illustration of the volume pulse method (top) and the pressure pulse method (bottom). Notice the difference in the sensor placement. Provided by G. Drzewiecki.

In the volume pulse method (Fig. 5-16), the successful recording hinges on the relationship between intravascular pressure distention and radial displacement. For a cylindrical uniform isotropic vessel, the relation is

$$\frac{dr}{dp} = \frac{3}{2} \frac{r(r+h)^2}{Eh(2r+h)} \tag{5-13}$$

where $r$ and $h$ are the radius and wall thickness, respectively. $E$ is the elastic modulus of the wall.

Thus, radial displacement ,$\Delta r$, due to a small change in arterial distending pressure, $\Delta p$, is

$$\Delta r = dr/dp \; \Delta p \tag{5-14}$$

Thus, the skin surface displacement is proportional to changes in arterial pressure. The skin surface is allowed to displace freely.

The pulse pressure method (Fig. 5-16), such as the tonometer is dependent on the interplays of contact stress, the deformation stress, and arterial pressure (which is actually a fraction of the contact stress). Drzewiecki et al. (1983) have shown that, in arterial tonometery, with arterial flattening, shear stress becomes negligible, compared with the normal stress in the arterial wall and skin, and uniform contact stress is developed over the transducer–skin interface. This is the ideal state for pulse recording with tonometry.

Arterial tonometry (Pressman and Newgard, 1963; Drzewiecki et al., 1983) for measuring BP is based on the principle that, when a pressurized blood vessel is partially collapsed by an external object, the circumferential stresses in the vessel wall are removed and the internal and external pressures are equal. Since tonometers are basically force transducers, they are useful only when applied to superficial arteries with solid bone backing (Fig. 5-17). Use of tonometer in the clinical setting has become increasingly popular, particularly in its application to the carotid (Chen et al., 1996) and the radial (Chen et al., 1998) arteries.

## 5.3. Blood Flow Measurements

### 5.3.1. ELECTROMAGNETIC FLOWMETER

Accurate measurement of blood flow lagged behind that of pressure for some years. Kolin (1936) introduced the now-popular electromagnetic flowmeter. It is based on Faraday's law of induction:

$$E = v \times B - J/\sigma_c \qquad (5\text{-}15)$$

where the induced electric field is $E$, in a conductor moving with a velocity, $v$, in a magnetic field intensity, $B$. $J$ is the current density and $\sigma_c$ is the conductivity (of blood). Figure 5-18 illustrates the principle. Bevir's (1971) virtual current theory, however, presents a more practical analysis.

Wyatt (1984) has reviewed blood flow and velocity measurement by electromagnetic induction. The cannular flowmeters with uniform field and point electrodes have the defect of a high degree of dependence on velocity distribution when they are not symmetric. The perivascular flowmeters have two defects: In addition to their sensitivity to velocity distribution, they are also sensitive to wall conductivity effects. The former can be reduced by using insulated- or multiple-electrodes, which improve the signal-to-noise ratio. Catheter-tip flowmeter (Mills, 1966; Kolin, 1967; Kolin et al., 1969) has the advantage that it is unaffected by the vessel wall. Boccalon et al. (1978) has devised a noninvasive electromagnetic flowmeter, which provides useful clinical applications.

### 5.3.2. DOPPLER VELOCIMETERS

Ultrasonic methods of measuring blood flow velocity are based on either the transmission or the reflection of ultrasound. Ultrasound propagation velocity through biological tissue is about 1560 m/s. Its associated wavelength can be easily calculated from

$$\lambda = c/f \qquad (5\text{-}16)$$

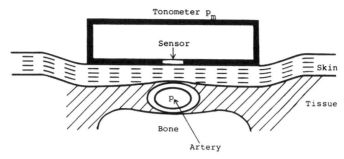

Fig. 5-17. Illustration of the principle of tonometry, similar to the pressure pulse method shown above, the area of contact and contact stress are critical for accurate recording. Provided by G. Drzewiecki.

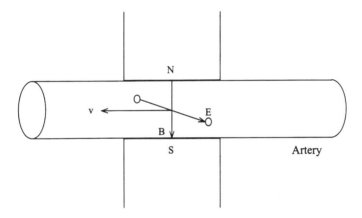

Fig. 5-18. Illustration of electromagnetic blood flow measurement principles. The moving conductor (blood with velocity, v) in a magnetic field (B) induces an electric motive force, and the potential (E) is picked up by the electrodes.

Typical diagnostic ultrasound utilizes frequencies in the range of 2–10 Mhz. Thus, the corresponding wavelengths are 0.78 and 0.156 mm, respectively. The ultrasound Doppler technique is based on the backscattering of ultrasound by red blood cells. Turbulence, therefore, increases the scattering. Two commonly used types are continuous-wave Doppler (CWD) and pulsed wave Doppler (PWD). In the CW mode, the Doppler-shifted frequency, $f_d$, of the backscattered ultrasound is:

$$f_d = \frac{2v \cos\theta}{c} \times f_0 \qquad (5\text{-}17)$$

where $v$ is the blood velocity, $\theta$ is the angle between the ultrasound beam and the centerline, and $f_o$ is the transmitted ultrasound frequency. In the PW mode, a velocity profile across the vessel can be obtained. Signal from cells scatters in a range at a depth of

$$z = \frac{ct_d}{2}$$

$$(5\text{-}18)$$

By pulsing the ultrasound beam, one can obtain range resolution along the beam. Generally, a short burst of ultrasound is transmitted with a repetition frequency, $f$. The backscattered signal is received and sampled after a time delay, $t_d$. Other applications of ultrasound can be found in, e.g., Reneman (1974) and Wells (1971).

Velocity profiles can also be obtained by the use of thermal-convection velocity sensors, such as hot-wire anemometers. Thermistors have been popular thermal velocity probes, mounted on either a catheter or a needle. These sensors have been applied to clinical settings (Roberts, 1972).

In general, Doppler-measured blood flow velocity compares well with that obtained by electromagnetic method (Figs. 5-19 and 5-20).

## 5.4. Thermodilution Measurement of Cardiac Output

The introduction of indicators to the circulatory system for the quantification of cardiac output (CO) has been used for some time and dye dilution has also been used for many decades. The principle of the indicator dilution method for measurement of cardiac output is illustrated in Fig. 5-21 (Geddes, 1984) in which an indicator of known mass is injected upstream. With the velocity of blood flow, the indicator is diluted, and its concentration is detected and sampled downstream. The amount of flow, $Q$, is calculated from the relation:

$$Q = \frac{m}{C_c \times t}$$

$$(5\text{-}19)$$

where $m$ is the mass of the injectate, $C_c$ is the concentration, and $t$ is time. Commonly used dyes are Evans blue and indocyanine green.

Thermodilution has become the most popular technique for monitoring cardiac output during routine clinical catheterization. The thermodilution technique was apparently first described by Fegler (1954) and became popular since its demonstrated use in humans by the groups of Swan et al., (1970), Ganz et al. (1971), and Forrester et al. (1972), with a single balloon-tipped flow-directed catheter. This method is illustrated in Fig. 5-22. Several investigators have evaluated the usefulness and accuracy of thermodilution (e.g., Weisel et al., 1975; Levett and Replogle, 1979; Kim and Lin, 1980; Bilfinger et al., 1982). Just as the Cournand catheter bears the name of its inventor for blood pressure measurement, the thermodilution catheter bears the name Swan-Ganz.

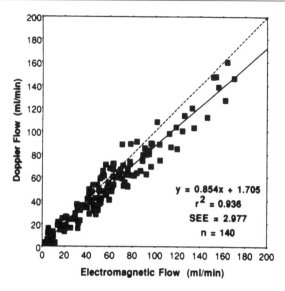

Fig. 5-19. Correlation of Doppler-ultrasound-measured blood flow velocity with that obtained by electromagnetic flowmeter. Good linear correlation is seen. Adapted with permission from Doucette et al. (1993).

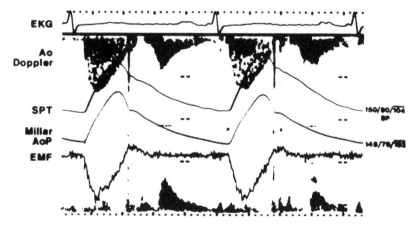

Fig. 5-20. Simultaneously measured aortic flows with the electromagnetic probe and Doppler velocity probe are shown. Noninvasive subclavian pressure pulse (SPT) is shown and compared to intravascular AoP waveform (Millar AoP). Adapted with permission from Marcus et al. (1994).

The thermodilution method is based on the Stewart-Hamilton principle, and is similar to other indicator dilution techniques. Stewart (1921) showed in experimental dogs that, if a known concentration of indicator is intro-

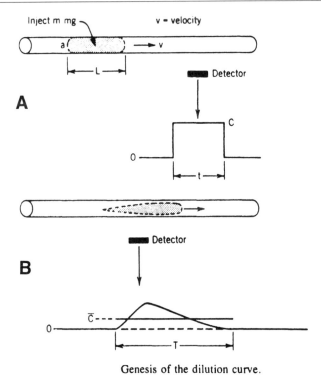

Genesis of the dilution curve.

Fig. 5-21. Principle of the dye dilution technique and the genesis of the dye dilution curve of concentration vs time. Adapted with permission from Geddes (1984).

duced into a flow stream and its temporal concentration is measured at a downstream site, then the volume flow can be calculated. The Stuart-Hamilton principle relates the flow ($Q$) to the mass ($m$) of indicator injected and the concentration ($c(t)$) of the indicator measured downstream at time, $t$:

$$Q = \frac{m}{\int_0^\infty c(t)dt} \qquad (5\text{-}20)$$

Thus, if the area under the concentration vs time curve is found, flow can be easily obtained. When applied to measuring cardiac output, however, the continuous pumping of the heart introduces the problem of recirculation. To overcome this, an exponential extrapolation of the concentration–time curve's descending limb is imposed, so that an approximation of the integral with the area under the curve is achieved.

Indicators that have commonly been used include Evans blue dye, Indocyanine green, and some radioactive isotopes, such as albumin [131]iodide. The advantage of the nontoxicity and affordability of repeated

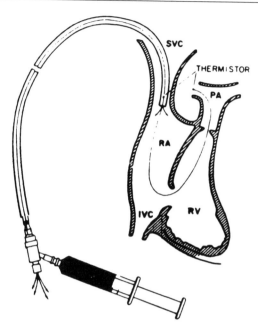

Fig. 5-22.Thermodilution method in man. The injection catheter is in the superior vena cava (SVC). The thermistor for measurement of indicator temperature is inside the injection catheter, 1–2 cm from the tip. The thermistor for measurement of blood temperature is in a main branch of the pulmonary artery (PA). RA and RV are right atrium and right ventricle, respectively. Adapted with permission from Ganz et al. (1971).

determinations within a short time-span makes cold solutions excellent choices as indicators. The advent of thermodilution has made cold saline and dextrose popular indicators. Typically, normal saline or isotonic dextrose (5%) in water is used as the injectate, either at 0°C or at room temperature. The most popular site of injection is the right atrium, and the sampling site is the pulmonary artery. By this choice of sites, the effect of recirculation is minimized. In this approach, a flow-directed, balloon-tipped catheter can be introduced into a vein (e.g., basilic vein in the arm) and, upon inflation of the balloon, the catheter is guided with the flow into the right atrium, the right ventricle, or the pulmonary artery. The exact site is normally confirmed with the pressure waveform recorded at the tip. The thermodilution catheter typically has a thermistor (thermal resistor) built in near the tip of the catheter, to monitor sampling site temperature. The faster the flow, the greater the temperature increase.

An example of the thermodilution method demonstrated by Ganz et al. (1971) is shown in Figs. 5-22 and 5-23, in which a 10 mL of cold (0.5–5°C) isotonic dextrose solution was injected into the superior vena cava of a

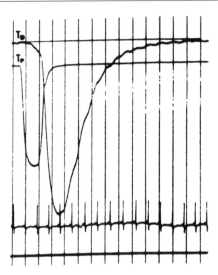

Fig. 5-23. Thermal curves recorded in a patient with normal circulation. Rewarming of the proximal thermistor ($T_p$) is rapid, and the thermal curve in the pulmonary artery has an exponential rewarming part. ECG is also shown at the bottom. Adapted with permission from Ganz et al. (1971).

patient with normal circulation. The injectate was delivered in 1–2 s. The area under the thermal curve was found by planimetry. This can now be obtained with an analog integrator or on-line with a digital computer.

For the thermodilution technique, the standard cardiac output determination in vivo is normally calculated from the following formula:

$$CO = \frac{V_i(T_b - T_i)S_iC_i60}{S_bC_b\int \Delta T_b(t)dt} \, F_c \qquad (5\text{-}21)$$

where $V_i$ = volume of the injectate in milliliters; $T_b$, $T_i$ = temperature of the blood and injectate, respectively; $S_b$, $S_i$ = specific gravity of the blood and injectate, respectively; and $C_b$, $C_i$ = specific heat of blood and injectate, respectively.

The ratio of $(S_iC_i):(S_bC_b)$ is 1.08 when 5% dextrose in water is used as an indicator. This ratio is 1.10 when normal saline is used. The specific gravity values for blood, dextrose and saline are 1.045, 1.018, and 1.005, respectively. The corresponding specific heat values for these solutions are 0.87, 0.965, and 0.997.

There is temperature differential between the site of injection and the delivery site where the injected solution begins mixing with blood. This temperature difference is dependent on several factors, including the rate of injection, the injected volume, the catheter injection lumen size, the length of the catheter between the two sites, the length of the catheter in blood, and the catheter material. For example, when 5 mL ice-cold saline is injected over 2 s, its temperature increases steadily through the catheter, which is already immersed in the blood stream. By the time the saline begins mixing with blood at the delivery site, e.g., in the right atrium, its temperature may be increased to 4–6°C. This, therefore, needs to be corrected. The correction factor, $F_c$, results from indicator heat loss along the catheter. $F_c$ is given as:

$$F_c = \frac{T_b - T_{id}}{T_b - T_i} \qquad (5\text{-}22)$$

where $T_{id}$ is the temperature of the injectate through the catheter at the delivery site. Ideally, the value of $F_c$ is 1.0, or the temperature at the injection site and delivery site is the same, or in other words, there is no heat loss through the catheter. In practice, for most thermodilution catheters, the correction factor, $F_c$ has been reported to be between 0.8 and 0.9. The accuracy of thermodilution has been verified against electromagnetic flow-meter and other established indicator dilution techniques. Thermodilution determined cardiac output has been shown to correlate well with the traditional dye dilution technique. This is shown in Fig. 5-24.

### 5.5. Vascular Ultrasound Dimension Measurement

Dimensions such as lengths have been measured with strain gages. These may be elastic, fine-wire, or solid-state. Mercury-in-silastic rubber, constantan, silicon, and germanium transducers are examples. They are based either on dimensional change or resistivity ($\rho_r$) change, i.e., the change in resistance ($\Delta R$) is derived from:

$$R = \frac{\rho_r L}{A} \qquad (5\text{-}23)$$

and

$$\frac{\Delta R}{R} = (1 + 2\sigma) \frac{\Delta L}{L} + \frac{\Delta \rho_r}{\rho_r} \qquad (5\text{-}24)$$

The first term on the right-hand side results from dimensional effect, and the second term to piezoresistive effect. A is cross-sectional area and L is the length of the strain gage wire. $\sigma$ is the Poisson ratio, defined in Eq. 2-15. Strain gage transducers can be applied to measure length, as well as pressure. In both cases, the resultant change in resistance is detected by a Wheatstone bridge circuitry.

An ultrasonic dimension gage has the advantage of high resolution, but also the disadvantage of more complex circuitry than strain gages. The

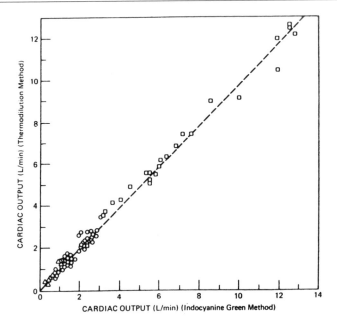

Fig. 5-24. Cardiac output determined by the thermodilution technique is plotted against dye dilution technique. Good linear correlation is obtained. Adapted with permission from Weissel et al. (1975).

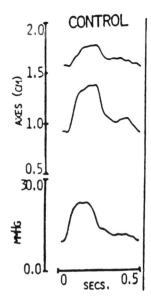

Fig. 5-25. Major and minor axes diameters of the pulmonary trunk measured by pairs of 3 MHz ultrasonic dimension gages. Bottom tracing is pulmonary pressure.

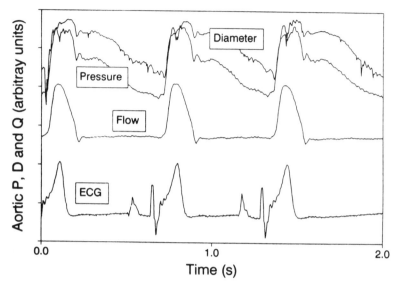

Fig. 5-26. Simultaneous recording of ultrasonic aortic diameter, aortic pressure, aortic flow, and ECG from a conscious instrumented dog. Provided by P. L. M. Kerkhof.

method requires a pair of piezoelectric transducers (e.g., barium titanate or lead zironate titantate, LTZ-5 MHz) either sutured or glued to the opposite sides of a vessel, for pulsatile diameter measurement. It is operated in the PW mode at $f = 1$ KHz. Figure 5-25 shows a typical recording of the main pulmonary trunk diameters (major and minor axes) with the ultrasonic dimension gages. Dynamic measurements of large-vessel diameter and wall thickness can be simultaneously recorded with an ultrasonic echograph. However, its limitation lies in boundary identification and resolution.

The small size of piezoelectric crystal ultrasonic dimension transducers allows their implantation for chronic and conscious animal studies. An example of this is shown in Fig. 5-26, in which simultaneously recorded ultrasonic aortic diameter, together with aortic pressure, aortic flow, and ECG, are obtained from a conscious instrumented dog. This allows on-line calculations of pressure–diameter relation, viscoelastic properties, and impedance, as well as wave reflection information.

## REFERENCES

Arzbaecher, R. C. and Novotney, R. L. Noninvasive measurement of the arterial pressure contour in man. *Bibl. Cardiol.* 31:63, 1973.
Bevir, M. Sensitivity of electromagnetic velocity probes. *Phys. Med. Biol.* 16:229–232, 1971.

Bilfinger. T. V., Lin, C.-Y., and Anagnostopoulos, C. E. In Vitro determination of cardiac output measurements by thermodiluation. *J. Surg. Res.* 33:409–414, 1982.

Boccalon, H., Candelon, B., Puel, P., Enjalbert, A., and Doll, H. Assessment of pulsatile blood flow by a noninvasive electromagnetic device. In: Dietlifich, E. B., ed., *Noninvasive Cardiovascular Diagnosis,* University Park Press, Baltimore, pp. 231–240, 1978.

Chen C.-H., Ting, C-T., Nussbacher, A., Nevo, E., Kass, D. A., Pak, P., Wang, S.-P., Chang, M.-S. and Yin, F. C. P. Validation of carotid artery tonometry as a means of estimating augmentation index of ascending aortic pressure. *Hypertension* 27:168–175, 1996.

Chen C-H., Nevo, E., Fetics, B., Pak, P. H., Yin, F. C. P., Maughan, W. L., and Kass, D. A.. Estimation of central aortic pressure waveform by mathematical transformation of radial tonometry pressure. *J. Am. Coll. Cardiol.* 32:1221–1227, 1998.

Cournand, A. and Ranges, H. A. Catheterization of the right auricle in man. *Proc. Soc. Exp. Biol. Med.* 46:462–466, 1941.

Doucett J. W., Gotto, M., Flynn, A. E., Austin, R. E., Jr., Hussaini, W., Hoffman, J. I. E. Effect of cardiac contraction and cavity pressure on myocardial blood flow. *Am. J. Physiol.* 265:H1342–1352, 1993.

Drzewiecki, G. M., Melbin, J. and Noordergraaf, A. The Korotkoff sound. *Ann. Biomed. Eng.* 17:325–359, 1989.

Drzewiecki, G. M., Melbin, J., and Noordergraaf, A. Noninvasive blood pressure recording and the genesis of Korotkoff sound. In: Shalak, R. and Chien, S., eds., *Handbook of Bioengineering*, McGraw-Hill, New York, 1987.

Drzewiecki, G. M. *Origin of the Korotkoff Sounds and Arterial Tonometry.* Ph. D. dissertation, University of Pennsylvania, Philadelphia, 1985.

Drzewiecki, G. M., Melbin, J., and Noordergraaf, A. Arterial tonometry: review and analysis. *J. Biomech.* 16:141–152, 1983.

Falsetti, H. L., Mates, R. E., Carroli, R. J., Gupta, R. L., and Bell, A. C. Analysis and corrections of pressure waveform distortion in fluid-filled catheter systems. *Circulation* 49:165–172, 1974.

Fegler, G. measurement of cardiac output in anesthetized animals by a thermodilution method. *Q. J. Exp. Physiol.* 39:153–164, 1954.

Forrester, J. S., Ganz, W., Diamond, G., McHugh, T., Chonette, D. W., and Swan, H. J. C. Hermodilution cardiac output determination with a single flow directed catheter. *Am. Heart J.* 83:306–311, 1972.

Forssmann, W. Die Sondierung des rechten Herzens. *Klin. Wochschr.* 8:2085, 1929.

Fry, D. L., Noble, F. W., and Mallos, A. J. An evaluation of modern pressure recording systems. *Circ. Res.* 5:40–46, 1957.

Ganz, W., Donoso, R., Marcus, H. S., Forrester, J. S., and Swan, H. J. C. A new technique for measurement of cardiac output by thermodiluation. *Am. J. Cardiol.* 27:392–396, 1971.

Geddes, L. A. *Cardiovascular Devices and Their Applications.* Wiley, New York, 1984.

Geddes, L. A. and Whistler, S. W. Error in indirect measurement with the incorrect size of cuff. *Am. Heart J.* 96:4–8, 1978.

Geddes L. A., Voelz, M., Combs, C., Reiner, D., and Babbs, C. F. Characterization of the oscillometric methods for measuring indirect blood pressure. *Ann. Biomed. Eng.* 10:271, 1982.

Geddes, L. A. *Handbook of Blood Pressure Measurement.* Humana, Clifton, NJ, 1991.

Geddes, L. A. and Baker, L. E. *Principles of Applied Biomedical Instrumentation.* Wiley, New York, 1989.

Hansen, A. T. Pressure measurement in human organisms. *Acta Physiol. Scand.* 19(Suppl. 68):1–227, 1949.

Hyatt, W. H. and Kemmerly, J. E. *Engineering Circuit Analysis.* McGrawHill, New York, 1978.

Karvonen M. J., Telivuo, L. J. and Jarniven, E. J. K. Sphygmomanometer cuff sizes and the accuracy of indirect measurement of blood pressure. *Am. J. Cardiol.* 13:688, 1964.

Kim, M. E. and Lin, Y. C. Determination of catheter wall heat transfer in cardiac output measurement by thermodilution. *Clin. Exp. Pharmacol. Physiol.* 7:383–389, 1980.

Kirkendall W. M., Feinleib, M., Freis, E. D., and Mark, A. Recommendations for human blood pressure determination by sphygmomanometers. *Hypertension* 3:510a, 1981.

Kolin, A. A new principle for electromagnetic catheter flowmeter. *Proc. Nat. Acad. Sci. USA* 63:357–363, 1969.

Kolin, A., Archer, J., and Ross, G. An electromagnetic catheter flowmeter. *Circ. Res.* 21:889–899, 1967.

Kolin, A. Electromagnetic flowmeter. The principle of the method and its application to blood flow measurement. *Proc. Soc. Exp. Biol. Med.* 35: 53–56, 1936.

Korotkoff, N. C. On the subject of methods of determining blood pressure. *Wien med. Wochenschr.* II:365, 1905.

Latimer, K. E. Transmission of sound waves in liquid-filled catheter tubes used for intravascular blood-pressure recording. *Med. Biol. Eng.* 6:29–42, 1968.

Levett, J. M. and Replogle, R. L. Thermodilution cardiac output: a critical analysis and review of the literature. *J. Surg. Res.* 27:392–404, 1979.

Levine S. R. True diastolic blood pressure. *New Engl. J. Med.* 304:362, 1981.

Li, J. K.-J., Melbin, J., and Noordergraaf, A. Pressure-gradient determination with sStandard laboratory transducers. *Proc. 13th Assoc. Adv. Med. Instrum.* 13:174, 1978.

Li, J. K.-J. and Kostis, J. B. Aspects determining accurate diagnosis and efficacy of catheterization. *Proc. 1st Int. Congr. Med. Instrum.* A07, 1984.

Li, J. K.-J. and Noordergraaf, A. Evaluation of needle-manometer and needle differential-manometer systems in the measurement of pressure differences. *Proc. 3rd NE Bioeng. Conf.* 5:275–277, 1977.

Li, J. K.-J. and Matonick, J. P. Site-specific performance requirements of catheter-transducer systems for accurate blood pressure measurements. *Proc. 33rd. Assoc. Adv. Med. Instrum.* pp. 81-82, 1998.

Li, J. K.-J., Van Brummelen, A. G. W., and Noordergraaf, A. Fluid-filled blood pressure measurement systems. *J. Appl. Physiol.* 40:839–843, 1976.

London, S. B. and London, R. E. Comparison of indirect blood pressure measurements (Korotkoff) with simultaneous direct bracial artery pressure distal to cuff. *Adv. Intern. Med.* 13:127–142, 1967.

Marcus R. H., Korcarz, C., McCray, G., Neumann, A., Murphy, M., Borow, K., et al. Noninvasive method for determination of arterial compliance using Doppler echocardiography and subclavian pulse tracings. *Circulation* 89:2688–2699, 1994.

Marey, E. J. *La Methode Graphique dans les Sciences Experimentales et Principalement en Physiologie et en Medicine.* Masson, Paris, 1885.

Matonick, J. P., and Li, J. K.-J. Noninvasive monitoring of blood pressure during hand-grip Stress induced vascular reactivity. *Proc. 34th. Assoc. Adv. Med. Instrum.* pp. 21, 1999.

Mauer, A. H. and Noordergraaf, A. Korotkoff sound filtering for automated three-phase measurement of blood rpessure. *Am. Heart J.* 91:584–591, 1976.

Mauer, A. H. and Noordergraaf, A. Korotkoff sound filtering for automated three-phase measurement of blood pressure. *Am. Heart J.* 91:584, 1976.

Melbin, J. and Spohr, M. Evaluation and correction of manometer systems with two degrees of freedom. *J. Appl. Physiol.* 27:749, 1969.

Mills, C. J. Catheter-tip electromagnetic flow probe. *Phys. Med. Biol.* 11:323–324, 1966.

Nilsson, J. W. *Electric Circuits.* Addison-Wesley, London, 1983.

Posey J. A., Geddes, L. A., Williams, H., and Moore, A. G. Meaning of the point of maximum oscillations in cuff pressure in the indirect measurement of blood pressure. *Cardiovasc. Res. Ctr. Bull. Houston* 8:15, 1969.

Pressman, G. L. and Newgard, P. M. Transducer for the continuous external measurement of arterial blood pressure. *IEEE Trans. Biomed. Electronics* 10:73–81, 1963.

Rabbany S. Y., Drzewiecki, G. M., and Noordergraaf, A. Peripheral vascular effects on auscultatory blood pressure measurement. *J. Clin. Monitoring* 9:9–17, 1993.

Ramsey, M. Blood pressure monitoring: automated oscillometric devices. *J. Clin. Monitoring* 7:56–67, 1991.

Ramsey, M. Noninvasive measurement of blood pressure. *Tech. Rep. Critikon* 1983.

Ramsey, M. Noninvasive automatic determination of mean arterial pressure. *Med. Biol. Eng. Comput.* 17:11–18, 1979.

Reneman, R. S. *Cardiovascular Applications of Ultrasound.* North-Holland, Amsterdam, 1974.

Riva-Rocci, S. Un nuovo sfigmomanometro. *Gazz. Med. Lombarda* 47:981, 1896.

Roberts, V. C. *Blood Flow Measurements.* Williams and Wilkins, Baltimore, 1972.

Rodbard, S., Rubinstein, H. M., and Rosenblum, S. Arrival time and calibrated contour of the pulse wave determined indirectly from recordings of arterial compression sounds. *Am. Heart J.* 53:205, 1957.

Rushmer, R. F. *Structure and Functions of the Cardiovascular System.* Saunders, Philadelphia, 1972.

Simpson J. A., Jamieson, G., Dickhaus, D. W. and Grover, R. Effect of size of cuff bladder on accuracy of measurement of indirect blood pressure. *Am. Heart J.* 70:208, 1965.

Stegall, H. F., Kardon, M. B., and Kemmerer, W. T. Indirect measurement of arterial blood pressure by Doppler ultrasonic sphygmomanometry. *J. Appl. Physiol.* 25:793–798, 1968.

Stewart G. N. Output of the heart in dogs. *Am. J. Physiol.* 57:27–50, 1921.

Weissel, R. D., Berger, R. L., and Hechtman, H. B. Measurement of cardiac output by thermodilution. *N. Engl. J. Med.* 292:682–284, 1975.

Wells, P. N. T. Clinical applications of ultrasonics. In: Watson, B. W., ed., *IEE Medical Electronics,* Peregrinus, London, 1971.

Wyatt, D. G. Blood flow and blood velocity measurement in vivo by electromagnetic induction. *Med. Biol. Eng. Comput.* 22:193–211, 1984.

# 6  Arterial Circulation and the Heart

## 6.1. Coupling of Heart and Arterial System

In hemodynamic terms, the function of the heart is to provide energy and to perfuse the organ vascular beds. For the heart to accomplish this efficiently, the arterial system plays a central role as the distributing conduits. Both the distributing arteries and the peripheral vascular beds present the load to the heart. Peripheral resistance has been popularly viewed in the clinical setting as the vascular load to the heart. This applies mostly to steady-flow conditions. This description is naturally inadequate, because of the pulsatile nature of blood flow, which remains throughout the microcirculation. Pulsatility implies that there is an oscillatory or pulsatile contribution to the vascular load to the heart.

We have seen that the input impedance of the arterial system has been used to represent this load, under steady-state conditions. This impedance contains components, such as the peripheral resistance, arterial compliance, and inertance. The impedance concept, though useful, is normally expressed in the frequency domain, and is thus difficult to interpret and use in the clinical setting, to relate directly to the arterial load. For this reason, peripheral resistance and arterial compliance, which can be obtained in the time domain, have been more popularly used, either individually or in combination, to describe the arterial load. Methods for their calculations are shown in Chapters 3 and 4. Change in arterial compliance or resistance, or both, therefore modifies the input impedance, and hence the arterial load.

Both decreased arterial compliance and increased peripheral resistance have been shown to be detrimental to cardiac function (Urschel et al.,1968; Li, 1987; Finkelstein et al., 1985; Kelly et al., 1992; Maruyama et al., 1993). Increased peripheral resistance is normally associated with an increase in mean arterial blood pressure and/or a decrease in mean blood flow. Arterial compliance is more related to arterial wall properties. A decreased arterial compliance is, therefore, associated with an increase in arterial wall stiffness or a reduction in intravascular lumen geometry. They

From: *Arterial Circulation: Physical Principles and Clinical Applications*
By: J. K-J. Li © Humana Press Inc., Totowa, NJ

increase the afterload to the heart, impede ventricular ejection, and increase the amount of external mechanical work that the heart must perform in order to provide adequate perfusion.

Several methods have been suggested to assess the coupling and the interaction of the heart and the arterial system. One such approach was proposed by Sunagawa et al. (1983,1985), based on experiments in isolated dog hearts, and later extended to humans (Kelly et al., 1992). An effective arterial elastance ($E_a$) was defined to represent the arterial system characteristics, although $E_a$ does not reflect the physical elastic properties of the arteries. Elastance as defined here, reflects only a system property. It does not equal the elastic properties of arteries. It is derived from the three-element windkessel model (Chapter 3), and is based on the assumption that the arterial system behaves linearly. As such, it is a steady-state parameter that incorporates peripheral resistance, arterial compliance, and characteristic impedance of the aorta, and systolic and diastolic intervals,

$$E_a = \frac{R_s}{[t_s + \tau(1 - e^{-t_d/\tau})]} \tag{6-1}$$

where $t_s$ and $t_d$ are systolic and diastolic periods, respectively. The diastolic pressure decay time constant is shown as before,

$$\tau = R_s C \tag{6-2}$$

$E_a$ has been approximated by the ratio of end-systolic pressure to stroke volume, or

$$E_a \approx P_{es}/SV \tag{6-3}$$

When the mean arterial pressure is used to approximate $P_{es}$, then $E_a$ can be easily estimated from

$$E_a \approx \bar{P}/V_s \tag{6-4}$$

Approximation of mean pressure to $P_{es}$ is good, when BP is in the normal range, under normal physiological conditions. It is a poor approximation in the case of strong vasoactive conditions, or when conditions affect arterial compliance or wave reflection.

Cardiac output is the product of stroke volume and heart rate,

$$CO = V_s f_h \tag{6-5}$$

where

$$f_h = 1/T \tag{6-6}$$

$T$ is cardiac period in seconds. The effective arterial elastance can be rewritten as

$$E_a \approx R_s/T \tag{6-7}$$

since $R_s$ is simply the ratio of mean arterial pressure divided by cardiac output.

Alternatively, when the diastolic aortic pressure decay time constant is long, compared with the diastolic period, or $\tau \gg t_d$, the denominator of Eq. 6-1 reduces to

$$t_s - \tau\,(1 - 1 - t_d/\tau) = t_s + t_d = T \tag{6-8}$$

where Taylor expansion is applied to the exponential term. When the assumption is also made that the peripheral resistance is much larger than the characteristic impedance of the aorta, or $R_s \gg Z_o$, then the effective arterial elastance (Eq. 6-1) becomes, again,

$$E_a \approx R_s/T \tag{6-9}$$

The effective arterial system elastance obtained in this manner is only dependent on the peripheral resistance and the cardiac period. It is totally independent of the elastic properties of the arterial system. In this treatment, arterial compliance is also ignored. The effective arterial system elastance, so defined, has the advantage that it is simple to use for the representation of the arterial load, but it has the disadvantage that the pulsatile nature of the arterial load is lost, e.g., compliance, characteristic impedance. When there is wave reflection or large change in compliance, this approximation works poorly.

In terms of ventricular function, a popular index used to describe its contractility is the maximal elastance of the ventricle. It is derived from the ventricular pressure–volume (P-V) relation (Suga et al., 1973). In this context, the ventricle is modeled with a time-varying compliance, $Cv(t)$, the inverse of which is the time-varying elastance, $E(t)$. Figure 6-1 illustrates the concept of $E(t)$ derived from the ratio of simultaneously measured ventricular pressure and volume. $E(t)$ increases from the beginning of systole to reach a maximum value, or $E_{max}$, at end-systole, and declines rapidly thereafter. The trajectory of $E(t)$ takes a finite amount of time, $t_{max}$, to reach $E_{max}$. With the infusion of epinephrine, which increases cardiac contractility, $E_{max}$ is much greater. This value is reached with shorter $t_{max}$. Thus, $E_{max}$ increases with increasing cardial contractility.

The concept of using $E_{max}$ as an index of cardiac contractility is more clearly seen in Fig. 6-2, which left ventricular pressure is plotted against left ventricular volume for several beats during control and during epinephrine. The P-V loop, follows an anticlockwise direction. It can be seen that the end-systolic points of the P-V loops lie on a straight line. This line intercepts the volume axis at $V_d$. At end-systole, the elastance ($E(t)$) slope is at its maximum and this defines $E_{max}$:

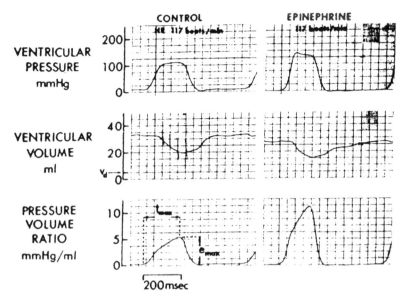

Fig. 6-1. LV pressure and volume and their instantaneous ratio obtained from isolated dog heart at control and during epinephrine infusion. The ratio increases from the beginning of systole to a maximum value of $E_{max}(e_{max})$ after a time, $t_{max}$, has elapsed. Adapted with permission from Suga et al. (1973).

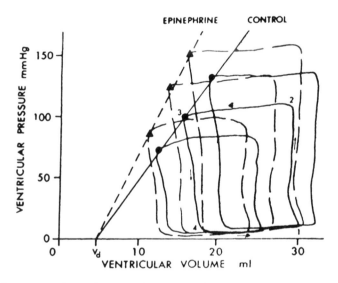

Fig. 6-2 Pressure-volume diagram of the LV defining ventricular elastance and $V_d$. The end-systolic P-V lines are drawn for contrl and epinephrine conditions. The slope representing the maximum elastance of the LV, or $E_{max}$, is increased during increased cardiac contractility with epinephrine. Adapted with permission from Suga et al. (1973).

$$E(t) = P(t)/[V(t) - V_o]; \quad E_{max} = P_{es}/(V_{es} - V_o) \qquad (6\text{-}10)$$

where $E_{max}$ is the maximum elastance of the ventricle, $V_{es}$ is the end-systolic volume, and $V_o$ is the dead volume, or the volume at which the ventricle no longer has the ability to develop pressure. Hence, it is the intercept on the volume axis, when the LV pressure is zero ($P_v = 0$). $V_o$ is difficult to measure experimentally or clinically. It has frequently been ignored in analyzing the interaction of the heart and the arterial system.

Neglect $V_o$ results in

$$E_{es} = P_{es}/V_{es} \qquad (6\text{-}11)$$

From the above relations, stroke volume has been used as a coupling variable for the ventricle and the arterial system, because it is the amount of blood ejected by the ventricle and received by the aorta per heartbeat. Despite its obvious limitations, the simple ratio of $E_a/E_{es}$ has been used extensively to characterize the interaction of the heart and the arterial system in conscious dogs (Little and Cheng, 1991), in exercising dogs (Hayashida et al., 1992) and in humans (Nichols et al., 1985; Kelly and Fitchett, 1992; Kelly, 1992a; Starling, 1993), and has been discussed recently by Hettrick and Warltier (1995). Figure 6-3 illustrates the steady-state coupling of the ventricle and the arterial system using the ratio of $E_a/E_{es}$.

It has been shown by Starling (1993) that the use of peripheral vasoactive agents, such as the potent vasoconstrictor, methoxamine (Li and Zhu, 1994), and the vasodilator, nitroprusside, do not alter the slope of the end-systolic P-V line, or $E_{es}$. But the slope of $E_a$ is increased with methoxamine and decreased with nitroprusside, as expected. As a result, the ratio of $E_a/E_{es}$ is altered, indicating changes in ventricle–arterial system coupling. With dobutamine, on the other hand, $E_a$ stays unaltered, but $E_{es}$ is increased, indicating changing cardiac contractility (Fig. 6-4). Thus, the coupling ratio $E_a/E_{es}$ can be altered by either changes in cardiac contractility or in arterial load. However, others showed that ventricular work and efficiency both remain nearly optimal, despite altered vascular loading (De Tombe et al., 1993).

The effects of alterations of windkessel arterial system parameters of characteristic impedance, arterial compliance, and peripheral resistance on the ventricular P-V relation under steady-state conditions (Fig. 6-5), has been investigated by Maughan et al. (1984), who found that the changes in arterial compliance and peripheral resistance have little effect on the slope of the end-systolic P-V relation. However, the shape and the trajectory of LV elastance are considerably altered.

There are other indices to cardiac performance, such as the pump function curve (Fig. 6-6) described by Van den Horn et al. (1984), and the

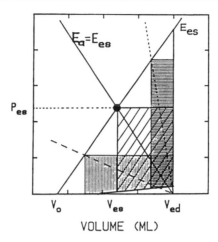

Fig. 6-3. Diagram defining the effective arterial elastance, $E_a$, showing its relation to the ventricular elastance, $E_{es}$. Adapted with permission from Sunagawa et al. (1984).

maximum velocity of cardiac muscle shortening by Krayenbuhl et al. (1978). There are also other indices to examine arterial system load behavior, such as the vascular overload concept proposed by Franklin et al. (1994,1997). Other aspects of the interaction, in terms of wave reflections and energetics, have also been investigated (Fitchett, 1991; Berger et al., 1995).

## 6.2. Dynamic Heart-Arterial System Interactions and the Concept of Dynamic Arterial Compliance

Dynamic interaction implies temporal relationship and instantaneous changes. This means that parameters used to interpret the interaction need to have a dynamic component that alters with time, within the cardiac cycle.

With varying systolic and diastolic blood pressures during a cardiac cycle, the compliance is also expected to vary continuously. This dynamic, time-varying pressure-dependent compliance property is incorporated in the recently developed nonlinear model of the systemic arterial system (*see* Chapter 3; Li et al., 1993a,1993b), shown on the right side of Fig. 6-7, in which the LV is represented by a time-varying compliance and a systolic resistance. The time-varying compliance is the inverse of time-varying elastance. The maximum elastance of the LV, or $E_{max}$, is defined by Eq. 6-10. The arterial system is defined by a nonlinear arterial system model that incorporates a pressure-dependent compliance element. Both time-varying compliance of the LV and the pressure-dependent compliance of the arterial system exhibit temporal dependence, and hence is dynamic in nature.

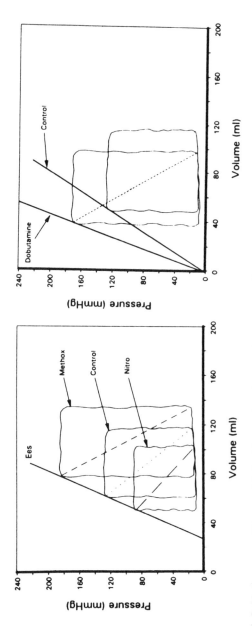

Fig. 6-4. P-V diagrams of the ventricle, illustrating the steady-state coupling of the ventricle and the arterial system, using the ratio of $E_a/E_{es}$. With methoxamine and nitroprusside infusions, the slope of $E_{es}$ is unchanged, but $E_a$ is altered. With dobutamine infusion, $E_{es}$ is increased, but $E_a$ is unchanged. Adapted with permission from Starling (1993).

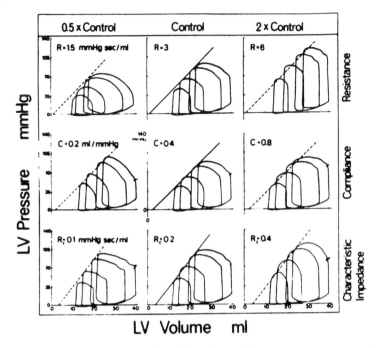

Fig. 6-5. Effects of alterations of windkessel arterial system parameters of characteristic impedance, arterial compliance, and peripheral resistance on the ventricular P-V relation under steady state conditions. Adapted with permission from Maughan et al. (1984).

In general, we found that reduced arterial compliance is associated with hypertension (Li et al., 1993a,1993b) and vasoconstriction (Zhu et al., 1992a,1992b). This reflects an increased dynamic component of the afterload to the heart. Zhu et al. originally established the temporal relationship between total systemic arterial compliance and BP within a single heartbeat, i.e., the arterial compliance varies continuously with BP in any given cardiac cycle. This has particular implications in terms of global heart–arterial system interaction. For instance, the pressure-dependent arterial compliance ($C(P)$) increases during the early systole, to facilitate ventricular ejection, but reaches a minimum at about end-systole. The dynamic elastance of the arterial system $E_{as}(t)$ (Li and Zhu, 1994), represented as the inverse of the pressure-dependent arterial system compliance, is shown in Fig. 6-8.

$$E_{as}(t) = 1/C(P) \qquad (6\text{-}12)$$

At end-systole, both time-varying arterial elastance and ventricular elastance are at their respective maximums ($E_{max}$) (Berger and Li, 1992;

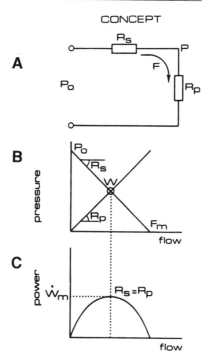

Fig. 6-6. The LV pump function curve concept, in which the ventricle has an internal source, $R_s$, resistance and ejects against an external resistance $R_p$. A working point (**B**) is established, based on the maximal power transfer (**C**). Adapted with permission from Van den Horn et al. (1984).

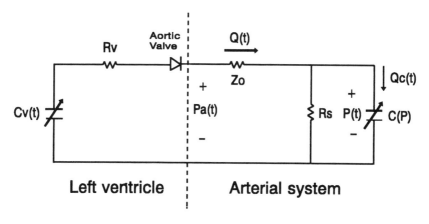

Fig. 6-7. Nonlinear model of the arterial system coupled to the LV. $Cv(t)$ = time-varying LV compliance, $R_v$ = systolic ventricular resistance, $Z_o$ = aortic characteristic impedance, $R_s$ = peripheral resistance, $C(P)$ = pressure-dependent or dynamic arterial compliance. $Pa(t)$ and $Q(t)$ are AoP and flow, respectively. Provided by Y. Zhu.

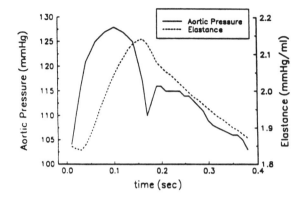

Fig. 6-8. Elastance of the arterial system, represented as the inverse of the pressure-dependent arterial system compliance, $C(P)$, defined by $E_{as}(t) = 1/C(P)$. The maximaum dynamic arterial elastance is reached at end-systole.

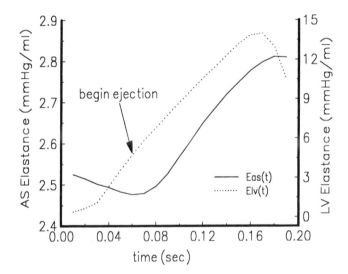

Fig. 6-9. Temporal relation of time-varying LV and arterial system elastances, demonstrating the dynamic interaction. Arterial system elastance is obtained from the pressure-dependent compliance ($E_{as}(t) = 1/C(P)$).

Fig. 6-9). The developing arterial elastance at systole reflects the time-varying compliance characteristics that are associated with active tension development of the arterial wall, as established for the ventricular muscle. This also demonstrates that the interaction of the heart and the arterial system is a dynamic one, particularly in systole. The arterial compliance thus bears a temporal, hence dynamic, relation to LV function.

## 6.3. Coronary Arterial Circulation

### 6.3.1. FUNCTIONAL IMPORTANCE OF THE CORONARY CIRCULATION

Coronary artery disease (CAD) has long been recognized as a leading cause of morbidity and mortality in industrialized nations. Although contributing factors are many, including hemodynamic and neurogenic factors, the consequential effects in structural alterations have been well documented. The arteriosclerotic nature of this disease has been known for centuries. This indicates the chronic and progressive nature of the disease, albeit the occurrence of coronary artery spasm. The first anatomical correlation between myocardial changes and CAD however, was apparently postulated only in the last century by Sir Richard Quain in 1850, whose suggestion of the connection between fatty softened heart and obstructed arteries has extended to this day. Identification of structural changes caused by CAD has led to the development in pathophysiological assessment of the disease. Its subsequent diagnostic interpretations and treatment have indeed dominated modern cardiovascular medicine.

The prevention of CAD has met with considerable difficulty, because about 40–60% of patients with sudden cardiac death or myocardial infarction present without previous symptoms. The absence of such warning symptoms has resulted in the so-called "silent-ischemia," which often involves coronary atherosclerosis.

Intervention to provide myocardial salvage has been popular, particularly thrombolysis, percutaneous transluminal coronary angioplasty (PTCA), coronary bypass surgery, o,r more recently, intravascular stent applications. For these techniques to be successful, the quantitative assessment of myocardial viability and local hemodynamic behavior need to be accurate. This is particularly true in the case of assessing the severity of coronary artery stenosis.

Assessment of functional severity of coronary stenoses had been limited to noninvasive techniques, such as stress electrocardiography, echocardiography, and radionuclide or myocardial scintigraphy. The other approach is to determine severity of isolated stenosis visualized with coronary angiography, which provides an estimate of the anatomical severity of stenosis. Noninvasive techniques cannot be used for immediate assessment of results of coronary interventions, when haziness of contours and wall disruption further impair the accuracy of conventional angiographic evaluation (Di Mario et al., 1994). Narrowing of the blood vessel defines the stenosis. The percentage occlusion is normally defined in terms of decrease in lumen diameter.

The amount of flow leaving the stenotic section is the same as that entering, conforming to that dictated by the equation of continuity:

$$Q = A_1 v_1 = A_2 v \tag{6-13}$$

Following Bernoulli's equation, the relation between the pressure drop and velocity gradient in the presence of stenosis can be written as

$$P_1 - P_2 = \tfrac{1}{2}\rho(v_2^2 - v_1^2) \tag{6-14}$$

For flow to occur through the stenosis, $P_1$ is necessarily greater than $P_2$, i.e. $P_1 > P_2$. It follows that the velocity at the stenosis section is faster, that is, $v_2 > v_1$.

The pressure gradient or the pressure drop across the stenosis, $\Delta P$, is given by

$$\Delta P = P_1 - P_2 \tag{6-15}$$

This has been shown to be dependent on the percentage occlusion. Figure 6-10 illustrates this, when the pressure drop is plotted against percent area stenosis. The pressure drop becomes significant only when the stenosis exceeds 70%. More detailed analysis of stenosis follows in Subheading 6.4.2.

### 6.3.2. ANATOMY AND PHYSIOLOGY OF THE CORONARY ARTERIAL SYSTEM

The coronary arteries and their main branches in humans are shown in Fig. 6-11. Chapter 7 deals with similarity analysis and comparative hemodynamics, but it suffices to state here that the global coronary anatomy, including the distribution of the major coronary arteries is very similar in many mammalian species. In general, intergroup differences are less pronounced than intragroup variations. There are two coronary arteries, right and left, arising, respectively, from the right anterior and left anterior aortic sinuses of Valsalva.

The left main coronary artery bifurcates into the anterior descending and circumflex branches. The anterior descending artery follows the anterior interventricular septum toward the apex, and is of variable length, terminating prior to, at, or beyond the apex. It gives rise to a number of ventricular branches. This artery also anastamoses with other branches, including the marginal and anterior ventricular branches of the left circumflex coronary artery and the posterior descending artery from the circumflex or right coronary artery (RCA). Other branches include the septal branches. The circumflex branch is largely an epicardial vessel, with anterior ventricular and atrial branches. Posteriorly, this artery communicates with the RCA either through the posterior descending or the marginal branches.

The RCA passes on the anterior side behind the pulmonary artery and follows the right atrioventricular groove to the right margin of the heart. In dogs and rabbits, it usually terminates here as the marginal branch; in pigs and humans, it usually reaches the posterior crux to become the posterior

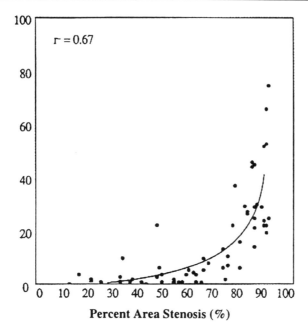

**Percent Area Stenosis (%)**

Fig. 6-10. Pressure drop across the stenosis is plotted against percent area stenosis. Notice that the magnitude of the pressure drop becomes significant only when area stenosis exceeds approx 70%. Adapted with permission from De Bruyne and Pijls (1995).

descending artery. Its branches include the atrial branches (which includes the branch to the sinoatrial [SA] node), right ventricular branches and a branch to the atrioventricular [AV] node. In general, the entire anterior and lateral LV is supplied by the left coronary branches, and the right ventricular free wall by the RCA. The most variable area of blood supply is the posterior region of the heart.

Besides the epicardial coronary arteries, there are also intramyocardial arteries. Although these arteries are not often visualized during routine coronary angiographic procedures, they are vital for the formation of critical anastomotic pathways and flow redistribution following obstruction of epicardial vessels. This is shown by a longitudinal section through the LV wall demonstrating branching of the two major types of intramyocardial vessels.

### 6.3.3. CORONARY COLLATERAL CIRCULATION

The importance of collateral circulation can be better appreciated when considering the coronary circulation in preserving and salvaging the myocardium under diseased conditions. Its relation to revascularization and angiogenesis has attracted particular interest in recent years. A collateral

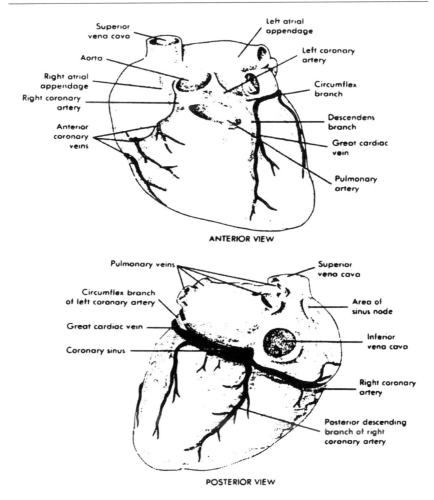

Fig. 6-11. Coronary arteries and their major branches shown in anterior and posterior views. Adapted with permission from Berne and Levy (1986).

circulation for an organ serves as an alternative to a major artery that has become nonfunctional, for instance, during an obstruction. Thus, a collateral channel is an initially unused pathway that is recruited only after failure of the original vessel to permit normal flows. However, the functional clinical significance of the coronary collateral circulation has continued to be debated, although extensive descriptions of the pathoanatomy and arteriography of this collateral circulation are available.

That a good coronary collateral circulation protects the myocardium has been recognized and demonstrated by some investigators. Collaterals may prevent myocardial infarction and thereby heart failure and result in improved survival.

### 6.3.4. Pressure-Flow Relationship in the Coronary Artery

The heart pumps blood to perfuse body organs, and to its own coronary vascular bed over a wide range of pressure and work demands. Ventricular contraction, with greatly increased intraventricular chamber pressure during systole, compresses the coronary vascular bed. This extravascular systolic compression inhibits its perfusion. The pulsatile energy stored in the compliant aorta allows the elastic recoil of this energy to facilitate perfusion of the myocardium during diastole. In diastole, with rapidly declining ventricular chamber pressure, the diastolic aortic pressure suffices to greatly perfuse the coronary arteries. Thus, aortic pressure serves as the perfusion to the coronary arteries. Coronary pressure–flow relation, however, is more complex than the one dictated by perfusion pressure and resistance (Klocke et al., 1985,1987). An example of the aortic pressure, left ventricular pressure and coronary flow relation is shown in Fig. 6-12.

The importance of coronary flow in terms of oxygen ($O_2$) delivery can be appreciated from the fact that oxygen extraction by the myocardial bed at rest can be as high as 75%, compared to 25% for the systemic vascular beds. Only through increased coronary blood flow (CBF) can elevated myocardial $O_2$ demands be met. The complex interaction of CBF, myocardial shortening, intramyocardial pressure, $O_2$ supply and demand, and the coronary vasculature can be readily appreciated. These anatomic, metabolic, and physiologic characteristics, in turn, determine the hemodynamic behavior of the coronary arteries. This has been utilized in the analysis of coronary artery stenosis and its coronary flow reserve. This has also generated methods for quantification of coronary artery abnormalities, such as the kinetics of radioactive tracers for perfusion and metabolic imaging, measurements of stenosis severity, the technical requirements of quantitative cardiac scanning, clinical manifestations of cardiac disease, and therapeutic interventions (Gould, 1974).

Coronary flow and flow reserve are both significantly compromised during CAD and stenosis. With progressive stenosis, the flow reserve is correspondingly reduced (Fig. 6-13), although there is a range in which autoregulation attempts to maintain flow. The autoregulation range lies between the lines of maximum vasodilation and maximum vasoconstriction.

Reactive hyperemia is a common phenomenon that is of particular importance to the analysis of the coronary circulation. Temporary coronary artery occlusion, even of very short duration, results in an immediate rapid rise in CBF out of proportion to the oxygen debt incurred during this temporary occlusion. The volume of blood repaid after the occlusion is typically 3–5× the volume deficit during the temporary occlusion. At maximum flow during this reactive hyperemia, myocardial arteriovenous $O_2$ difference narrows, indicating that the myocardial $O_2$ extraction is less

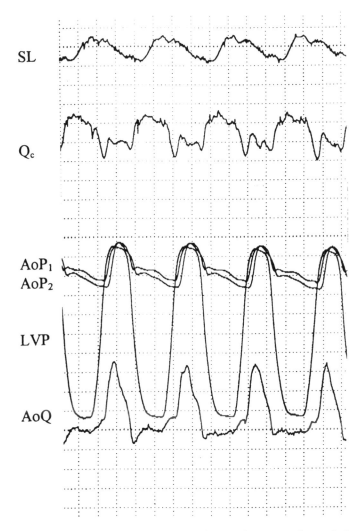

Fig. 6-12. AoP, LV pressure, segment length (SL), and coronary flow relations. AoP serves as the pulsatile perfusion pressure. Majority of coronary arterial flow ($Q_c$) occurs in diastole.

compared to the control resting flow conditions prior to reactive hyperemia. In other words, adequate $O_2$ is available to the myocardium, but is not extracted during the elevated flow after release of the occlusion.

The increase in CBF is just enough to compensate for the $O_2$ debt following temporary maintenance of the perfusion with deoxygenated blood. Thus, it is not just the lack of $O_2$ during occlusion that stimulates this disproportionate increase in coronary flow. Various mechanisms have been

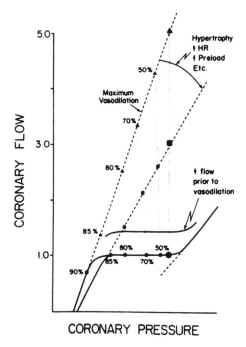

Fig. 6-13. Coronary flow reserve (CFR) and autoregulation curves. In CAD patients, the maximum vasodilation line is shifted right and lower, and the factors influence this shift are shown. In significant coronary arterial stenosis, CFR, shown as the difference between the maximum vasodilation (dashed) and autoregulation (solid) lines, is reduced with increased percentage stenosis. Adapted with permission from Klocke (1987).

proposed as the basis for this reactive hyperemia, including high shear forces that cause release of endothelial releasing factor, and the role of $O_2$ tension. Figure 6-14 below is a schematic diagram of this reactive hyperemia process, both as a result of occlusion and perfusion with deoxygenated blood. An experimentally recorded reactive hyperemic response in the left circumflex coronary artery is shown in Fig. 6-15. As with experimental stenosis, the mean flow during reactive hyperemia is a function of the lumen diameter (Fig. 6-16).

The effect of reactive hyperemia can often be estimated from pressure gradient recordings within coronary arteries. Figure 6-17 illustrates this. The ascending AoP is the main perfusion pressure, and when a distal coronary artery pressure is measured, their difference provides the pressure gradient, which is related to flow. Under normal conditions, there is a pulsatile pressure gradient and a small mean pressure difference between the two pressures. In hyperemia, the differences in both pulsatile pressure gradient and mean pressure become significantly large.

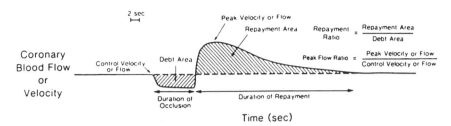

Fig. 6-14. Schematic diagram of reactive hyperemic flow response. After a brief occlusion, there is a significant increase in blood flow during the repayment period. The repayment ratio is an indication of the extent of reactive hyperemia. Adapted with permission from Marcus (1983).

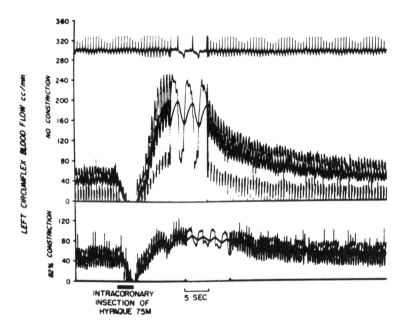

Fig. 6-15. Experimental recording of reactive hyperemia in the left circumflex coronary artery after injection of Hypaque with no constriction (upper tracing), and with 82% diameter constriction (lower tracing). Impairment in hyperemic response during stenosis in both phasic and mean (heavy line) flows are clearly seen. Adapted with permission from Gould et al. (1974).

Because of the clinical implications of myocardial ischemia caused by vessel obstruction, particularly, stenosis, quantitative hemodynamic analysis of the coronary circulation is of particular importance. There have been numerous studies on the phasic flow relations in the epicardial coronary arteries and the effect of extravascular systolic compression on coronary

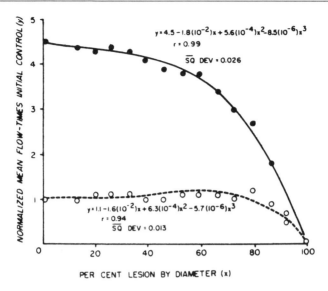

Fig. 6-16. Normalized mean flow times initial control plotted against percent diameter lesion for control (dashed line) and reactive hyperemia (solid line) conditions. Adapted with permission from Gould et al. (1974).

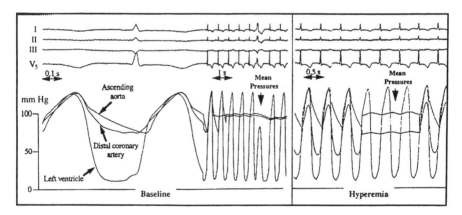

Fig. 6-17. Simultaneously recorded ascending AoP (*Pa*), LV pressure (*Pv*), and distal coronary artery pressure (*Pdca*) waveforms, showing dependency of a translesional pressure gradient on flow in a patient with obstructive proximal coronary artery. Notice the large pulsatile pressure gradient and mean pressure difference between *Pa* and *Pdca* during hyperemia (right). Adapted with permission from De Bruyne and Pijls (1995).

arterial flow, fewer studies have quantified the characteristics of phasic coronary inflow into the myocardium. For this latter perfusion, it is necessary to evaluate the phasic BF velocity in the distal coronary artery, since proximal coronary arterial flow may differ from the distal flow because of the effect of the variable compliance in epicardial arteries. Chilian and Marcus (1984) used high-frequency, pulsed ultrasound Doppler velocimeter to characterize the velocity waveform in distal coronary arteries, and concluded that the amount of flow in systole is decreased by more than half and the amount in diastole is increased by 20%, compared with the flow in the proximal coronary artery and that the mid-systolic flow is retrograde. Indeed, retrograde perfusion has been considered an important aspect of maintaining normal coronary perfusion.

### 6.3.5. MEASUREMENT OF CORONARY ARTERY PRESSURE AND FLOW

There are several methods of measuring coronary pressure and flow. The relative difficulty in the quantification of the hemodynamics of CBF has initiated the development of novel experimental techniques and devices. Quantitative coronary angiography, for instance, is now commonplace. Determination of pressure–flow characteristics of controlled, variable coronary stenoses in intact, unanesthetized, chronically instrumented animals, as well as acute, open-chest experiments in anesthetized dogs, have also been performed by several investigators. In addition to catheter-tip pressure measurement, an appropriately sized, perivascular electromagnetic flow transducer has been employed for flow determination in vivo.

Regional myocardial perfusion in humans in the past has included thermodilution and the gas clearance method, as well as radioactive microspheres, although this latter technique is mostly used in experimental animals. Modern use of Doppler techniques, positron-emission tomography and digital subtraction angiography are now commonplace. Recently, techniques employing magnetic resonance imaging and contrast echocardiography, however, permit precise measurement of perfusion in different layers of the LV myocardium, without cardiac catheterization (Marcus et al., 1983). Doppler flow velocity measurements for the coronary circulation are now most commonly done using a Doppler guide wire (Fig. 6-18). The guide wire is flexible and steerable with a ultrasonic (e.g., 12 MHz) piesoelectric transducer mounted at its tip. The transducer produces a broad beam (20° divergence angle) ultrasonic signal with an estimated sample volume of 2.25 mm diameter at a gated range depth of 5 mm. It can be used to cross a stenosis and guide an angioplasty balloon for dilation purposes (Segal et al., 1992). Commercially available Doppler systems calculate and display on-line several spectral variables, including instantaneous and time-averaged peak velocities and mean flow velocity, as well as diagnostic indices, such as coronary flow reserve. Reduced flow with stenosis can be easily appreciated from the pressure–velocity tracings shown in Fig. 6-19.

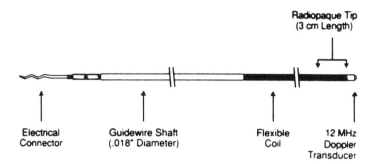

Fig. 6-18. Intravascular Doppler recording of blood flow velocity in a coronary artery with a guide wire. The guide wire has a 12-Mhz piezoelectric broad-beam Doppler transducer mounted on its tip. Adapted with permission from Segal et al. (1992).

In conjunction with flow measurements, a pressure sensor located about 2 cm proximal to the flexible tip of a 0.018-in. guide wire is commonly used. Commercially available systems have been validated regarding signal transfer characteristics, linearity and frequency response, as discussed in Chapter 5. The fractional flow reserve, $FFR_{myo}$, is defined, for a coronary artery as the ratio between maximum-achievable CBF to its dependent myocardium and the hypothetically maximum-achievable CBF to that same region, if the supplying artery is completely normal. This index has been used to determine the safety of deferral of PTCA of angiographically intermediate, but functionally nonsignificant, stenosis. A deferral on the basis of an $FFR_{myo} \geq 0.75$ has been regarded as safe.

## 6.4. Hemodynamics and Modeling of the Coronary Circulation

### 6.4.1. THE WATERFALL HYPOTHESIS AND CORONARY PRESSURE-FLOW ANALYSIS

The vascular waterfall model has been proposed (Downey and Kirk, 1975) as a basis for understanding the complex hemodynamics of the coronary arterial system (Sideman and Beyar, 1987). According to this model, there are two principal components that contribute to coronary resistance: the intravascular and extravascular components. The intravascular component results from smooth muscle tone in the coronary walls, and is determined by the diameter of the patent coronary vessels, which is under the influence of autoregulation and of the cardiac nerves. The extravascular component is derived from outside the coronary vessels and is the result of mechanical deformation of the coronary vessels, as the heart contracts and relaxes. There is a gradient in the extravascular resistance, and pressure development in the ventricular chamber was found to be the

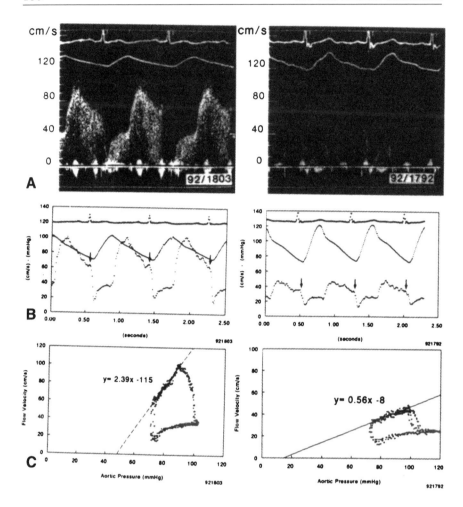

Fig. 6-19. (**A**) Simultanoeusly measured coronary pressure and Doppler velocity during maximum hyperemia in a left circumflex artery and in a left anterior descending coronary artery distal to a 56% diameter stenosis. (**B**) ECG, AoP and flow velocity as in A. Arrows indicate beginnning of contraction. (**C**) Flow velocity–pressure loops showing reduced slope in stenosis. Adapted with permission from Di Mario et al. (1994).

primary determinant of this gradient. Measurements of this gradient have shown that the highest pressure is at the subendocardium (this pressure is at least equal to ventricular pressure, and may exceed it), and there is near-zero pressure at the subepicardium.

The effect of this tissue pressure in reducing coronary flow has been modeled by the formation of vascular waterfalls for the coronary bed. The waterfall equations describe flow as a discontinuous function of resistance, arterial pressure, venous pressure and tissue pressure. When tissue pressure exceeds arterial pressure, the vessel is collapsed and flow is zero. When tissue pressure is less than venous pressure, flow is proportional to the arterial-venous pressure difference. When tissue pressure is between arterial and venous pressure, however, partial collapse of the vasculature causes flow to be proportional to the arterial pressure-tissue pressure difference. The complicating factor in the heart is that tissue pressure varies both spatially and temporally.

The waterfall model predicts that a unique pressure–flow curve exists for the coronary artery of a beating heart. This curve is straight above the peak tissue pressure and convex to the perfusion pressure axis below that peak pressure. In cardiac arrest, all tissue pressure is removed, and this causes the pressure–flow curve to become straight and to shift upward. These curves were proven correct from experiments performed on open-chest dog models. The model described above was found incapable of duplicating the coronary flow profile seen at the coronary ostium.

Coronary pressure–flow relationship has been analyzed by many investigators (Eng et al., 1982; Hoffmann, 1984; Bellamy and O'Benar, 1985; Li, 1987; Hoffmann and Spaan, 1990; Goto et al., 1996). Some have included coronary vascular capacitance as part of the coronary vascular impedance (Canty et al., 1985; Van Huis et al., 1987; Mates, 1988; Dai and Li, 1998; Frasch et al., 1998).

The waterfall model can partly explain the impediment of coronary blood flow in systole. It cannot explain the retrograde flow (Spann, 1981a,1981b). An intramyocardial pump concept was suggested, as a consequence of flow changes caused by intramyocardial compliance, in addition to flow changes caused by resistance alone. Thus, intramyocardial pump models were proposed (Rabbany et al.,1989). One such model is shown in Fig. 6-20, from Olsson et al. (1992), in which the phasic coronary flow is the resultant of two flow components. One results from arterial-venous pressure difference, the other is from intramyoardial pump, retrograde for arterial flow and forward for the venous flow (Beyar et al., 1993).

Bruinsma et al. (1988) have proposed a model similar to of Downey's waterfall model, but one that takes into account the structural connectedness of the microvessel with myocardial tissue. In both models microvessels can collapse, in the waterfall model, the vessel collapse occurs instantaneously and very locally (in theory, at an infinitely small spot). In Bruinsma's model of the coronary circulation based on pressure dependence of coronary resistance and compliance, such a local collapse does not occur, resulting in more homogeneously spread volume variations of vessels, and these variations require time to occur. In this model, the LV wall is subdivided (arbitrarily) into eight layers, from the endocardium to

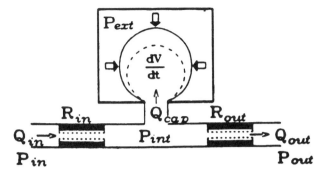

Fig. 6-20. Intramyocardial pump model. Two flow components, one resulting from arterial-venous pressure difference, the other from intramyocardial pump, are shown. Arrows indicate direction of pressure change, which results in a change in volume (compliance effect), the rate of change of which is flow. Adapted with permission from Olsson et al. (1992).

the epicardium, and the vasculatures of each of these layers is represented by an arteriolar, a capillary, and a venular compartment in series. Each compartment is compliant and hydrodynamically resistive.

In the above model, the inflow ($Q_{in}$) and outflow ($Q_{out}$) of a compartment are determined by the distribution of hydrostatic pressures :

$$Q_{in} = (P_p - P_c)/R \qquad (6\text{-}16)$$

and

$$Q_{out} = (P_c - P_d)/R \qquad (6\text{-}17)$$

The model described above predicts the pressure–flow relationships for the coronary circulation, and shows that models that contain fixed resistance and capacitance may seriously underestimate intramyocardial capacitance effects and characteristic time constants for pressure-induced resistance changes. Reneman and Arts (1985) have assessed the dynamic capacitance of epicardial coronary arteries from in vivo measurements in dogs. Dynamic capacitance is defined as the ratio of the increment in volume to the increment in pressure for a rapid pressure change. They calculated this value from the volume stiffness (derived from the pressure wave front velocity) and the volume of the arteries. They found the dynamic capacitance of the RCA, the anterior descending and circumflex branches of the LCA at an arterial pressure of 13.3 kPa and a frequency between 7 and 30 Hz, to be 0.0024 ± 0.0013, 0.0062 ± 0.0028, and 0.0079 ± 0.0035 mL/kPa (mean ± SD), respectively.

A number of models based on the waterfall mechanisms or intramyocardial capacitance, or a combination of them have been reported to explain

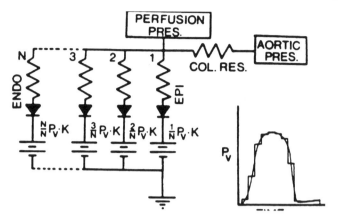

Fig. 6-21. Waterfall-mechanism-based model used to simulate pressure-flow relations. Adapted with permission from Downey and Kirk (1975).

coronary pressure–flow relation. Downey and Kirk (1975) proposed one such simple model, in which the rise and fall of intramyocardial pressure is simulated by making local tissue pressure proportional to ventricular pressure (Fig. 6-21). Tissue pressure is determined by multiplying ventricular pressure by appropriate coefficients. The coefficient increases from near zero at epicardium to unity at endocardium. The coefficient K determines the actual magnitude that the tissue pressure achieves at the endocardium. Collateral circulation, as in many studies, is represented by resistances in parallel. The drawback in this model is that capacitance effect is neglected.

A model that is used to explain the input impedance of the coronary circulation was proposed by Canty et al. (1985), and is shown in Fig. 6-22. Resistance and capacitance in parallel, and with viscoelastic properties, are incorporated in two models to predict the impedance behavior during intact and vasodilated conditions. The advantage of the model is that it allows quantification of the effect of capacitance (Mates, 1988; Mates and Judd, 1993).

A mathematical model that contains fixed resistances and capacitance has been proposed by Holenstein and Nerem (1990) on parametric analysis of flow in the intramyocardial circulation. In this model, shown in Fig. 6-23, the intramyocardial vascular bed is represented by three layers, each consisting of a simple three-parameter windkessel model with one constant capacitance, C, and two constant resistances, $R_1$ and $R_2$. This model has an obvious limitation: The entire coronary system has been lumped together, with a myocardium modeled only by three parallel layers and physical properties represented by a set of constant resistances and a single

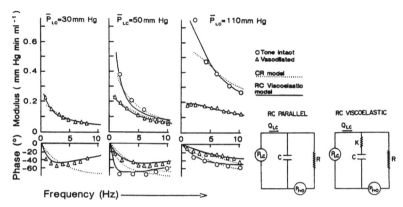

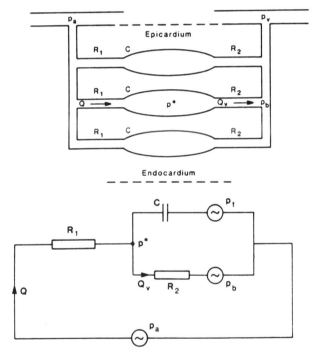

Fig. 6-22. Measured input impedance and impedances obtained from a parallel resistance–capacitance model (dashed lines) and the viscoelastic model (solid lines) for tone intact (open circle) and vasodilated (closed circle) beds. Adapted with permission from Canty, 1985.

Fig. 6-23. Mechanical model (top) and electrical analog (bottom) of the coronary microcirculation. Three-element windkessel model is incorporated here with a constant capacitance, $C$, and two constant reistances $R_1$ and $R_2$. The arterial ($P_a$), venous ($P_v$), tissue ($P_t$), and back pressures are also shown. $P^*$ is intracoronary pressure. Adapted with permission from Holenstein and Nerem (1990).

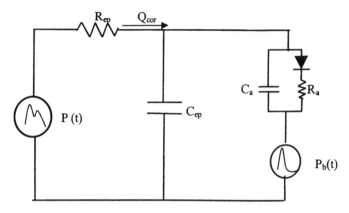

Fig. 6-24. Analog model of the coronary circulation for more description of coronary pressure–flow relation. Perfusion pressure, $Pf(t)$, and back pressure, $Pb(t)$, are shown with epicardial resistance ($R_{ep}$) and capacitance, and arterial resistance ($R_a$) and capacitance ($C_a$). Provided by J. Dai.

capacitance. This simple model, however, allows prediction of the general waveform shape and gross features of the system.

Quantification of the effect of ventricular contraction on coronary flow (e.g., Krams et al., 1989a,1989b) through modeling, has received considerable attention. For instance, Zinemanas et al. (1993) examined the effect of myocardial contraction on CBF and Vis et al. (1995,1997) developed a model to quantify coronary pressure–flow relations during systole and diastole, when the coronary artery is embedded in cardiac muscle.

A recently proposed model of the coronary circulation by Dai and Li (1999) is shown in Fig. 6-24. This model contains the required elements to sufficiently describe pressure-flow relations more completely: time-dependent perfusion pressure and back pressure, epicardial resistance and capacitance, and arterial capacitance and resistance. This model has been shown to predict measured pulsatile CBF waveforms accurately.

### 6.4.2. Stenosis-Related Coronary Hemodynamics

In coronary artery stenosis, resting CBF and regional flow distribution remain normal, despite progressive, relatively severe coronary artery narrowing. In fact, with up to approx 65–75% diameter narrowing, progressive coronary stenosis has no effect on resting coronary flow and causes no distal compensatory vasodilatation (Gould, 1974). Although the pressure-flow characteristics of coronary artery stenosis in vivo are mostly determined by the hemodynamic behavior of, and interaction with, the distal coronary vascular bed, it is not the compensating distal arteriolar vasodilatation that maintains this normal resting flow. The real explanation may be found in the relation between resting coronary vascular tone, or resistance, $R_t$, and the resistance of the proximal coronary stenosis, $R_{st}$, in series with the vascular bed.

The resting flow $Q$, in a model artery, is determined by the relation

$$Q = \frac{\Delta P}{R_{st} + R_b}$$ (6-18)

where $\Delta P$ is the total pressure gradient

Because normal resting coronary vascular resistance, $R_b$, is very high (four to five times its minimum resistance in the maximally vasodilated state), the proximal stenosis must be severe before its resistance approximates $R_t$, and begins to reduce resting flow. Thus, the coronary vascular system is normally a low-flow, high-resistance system at rest and is ideally suited to meet increased work demands by increasing flow. This high-resistance system is the reason why atherosclerosis is a clinically silent disease until it is anatomically severe and advanced, when angina pectoris appears. This also means that resting coronary flow is an insensitive and poor measure of stenosis severity, thus necessitating the need for alternate measures of stenosis severity, as will be considered in the next subheading

Stenosis characteristics have been studied both in vivo and in vitro. The coronary circulation has been considered as a series combination of a pulsatile pressure source (representing the aortic input pressure) and a time-varying distal resistance simulating the impediment of coronary flow during myocardial contraction. The circulation itself has been modeled in the maximally vasodilated state, since vasodilatation occurs as a physiological response to compensate for the loss in perfusion pressure caused by an arterial obstruction. The effect of a stenosis is thus reflected by a pressure loss and a decrease in flow. In vitro findings have generally resulted in possible clinical implications for the in vivo situation in which periodic motion of the normal wall circumference opposite an eccentric plaque may lead to fissuring or tearing of the intima. Also, because the fluid dynamics of a partially compliant stenosis may change continuously during the diastolic part of the cardiac cycle as the result of a passive change in the stenotic lumen area, the validity of hemodynamic characteristics based on angiographic dimensions or extrapolations over a wide range of flow rates should be treated with caution.

A method of hemodynamically characterizing the severity of coronary artery stenosis is important to the systematic or statistical evaluation of their effects in vivo. As has been pointed out earlier, for a geometrically fixed stenosis, pressure gradients across the stenosis are variable, and depend on flow, and, as such, cannot be used alone to quantify the effect of stenosis. Stenosis resistance has been evaluated as a means of characterizing stenoses hemodynamically (Gould, 1974). Stenosis resistance ($R_{st}$) has been defined as

$$R_{st} = G/Q \tag{6-19}$$

where $G$ is the mean reduction in pressure or gradient across the constriction, and $Q$ is the mean flow through it. But, because of the use of mean values, this variable was found to be misleading as a measure of stenosis severity.

As an alternative, the mean pressure gradient–flow relation during hyperemia has been used to quantify the hemodynamic severity of stenoses, for purposes of correlating them with compensatory changes of the distal coronary vascular bed. The slope of the pressure gradient–flow relation during hyperemia increases during modest anatomic stenosis, stenosis resistance remains normal.

With the introduction of miniaturized pressure and Doppler sensors with guide wire technology, measurement of the poststenotic flow velocity and pressure has been made possible in the catheterization laboratory. Based on these simultaneous measurements of transstenotic pressure gradient and flow velocity, DiMario et al. (1994) assessed the feasibility and clinical usefulness of different indices of stenosis severity. The indices were calculated on the basis of quantitative coronary angiography, Doppler flow velocity and pressure guide wire measurements. The transstenotic pressure gradient, $\Delta P$ (in mmHg), can be calculated from QCA measurements using the following equation:

$$\Delta P = \frac{8\pi\mu L}{1.33\,A_s^2}\,Q + \frac{k_e\rho}{0.266}\,[(1/A_s) - (1/A_n)]^2\,Q^2 \tag{6-20}$$

where $\mu$ is the dynamic blood viscosity in Poise (assumed equal to 0.03), $L$ the length of the stenosis in mm, $A_n$ the cross-sectional area of the normal reference segment in mm$^2$, $A_s$ the minimal cross-sectional area of the stenotic segment in mm$^2$, $Q$ the mean CBF in mL/s, $\rho$ the blood density in g/mL (assumed equal to 1.05), and $k_e$ the expansion coefficient used to correct for entrance effect.

### 6.4.3. CORONARY FLOW RESERVE

Coronary flow reserve (CFR) is an index often used for evaluating coronary stenosis, and has been defined as the ratio between maximal flow, $Q_M$, e.g., obtained at the peak effect of an injected vasodilator like adenosine, dipyridamole, or papavarine, and at baseline conditions, $Q_R$, i.e.,

$$CFR = Q_M/Q_R \tag{6-21}$$

This defines the capacity of coronary vasculature to increase its blood flow in accordance with myocardial $O_2$ demand.

Another common means is to obtain CFR from the hyperemic response. For instance, to obtain the flow reserve ratio in the vascular bed perfused by the circumflex coronary artery, one must first measure the circumflex blood flow at resting condition and the hyperemic response after a brief occlusion. The CFR is then:

$$CFR = Q_{MCFX}/Q_{RCFX} \qquad (6\text{-}22)$$

or the ratio of peak hyperemic circumflex artery blood flow to the resting circumflex flow. This approach has been employed, for example, by Ohtsuka et al. (1994).

Animal experiments have shown that measurement of impairment in maximal coronary flow is the ideal method to determine functional severity of stenosis, but it must also be pointed out that CFR is influenced by the hemodynamic conditions at the time of measurement, including heart rate and aortic pressure. The dynamic response of the coronary circulation to changes in heart rate has also been studied with system analysis techniques by Dankelman et al. (1989a,1989b). Also, several pathologic conditions, such as cardiac hypertrophy, myocardial scarring, diabetes, hypercholesterolemia, and systemic hypertension, induce more permanent changes of the hyperemic pressure–flow relationship. In these conditions, stenosis severity is overestimated if the low flow during maximal vasodilation is attributed to high resistance across the stenosis.

An alternative approach has been to estimate the stenosis flow reserve, which has been described as a single integrated index of stenosis severity, based on measurements of stenosis geometry, transstenotic pressure gradient and maximal flow increase under standardized conditions. However, as shown by DiMario et al. (1994), there is poor correlation between estimated stenosis flow reserve and measured CFR. FFR is another index that has been used to quantify stenosis severity, and is calculated as

$$FFR_{cor} = \frac{P_d - P_w}{P_a - P_w} \qquad (6\text{-}23)$$

where $P_d$ is the poststenotic coronary pressure, $P_a$, the mean arterial pressure, and $P_w$, the coronary wedge pressure. As can be seen from the equation for this ratio, measurements are necessary for arterial, distal coronary, and central venous pressures during maximum arteriolar vasodilation.

## 6.5. Myocardial Function and Arterial System Load

The study of pressure-dependent behavior of arterial compliance or vascular stiffness is important, because of its relevance to many cardiovascular diseases, some of which are result from alterations in the mechanical properties of the vessel wall and vascular states, as in the cases of hypertension and atherosclerosis (O'Rourke et al., 1970; Safar et al., 1984). In hypertension for instance, the increased pressure is always associated with a reduced arterial compliance (Simon et al., 1992; Hayoz et al., 1992; Meister et al., 1992). Reduced compliance impedes ejection, and is detrimental to normal LV function. A decreased compliance can occur as a consequence of an elevated arterial pressure and that an increased BP may result from decreased compliance as a result of alterations in vessel wall properties.

Both decreased arterial compliance and increased peripheral resistance are detrimental to ventricular function (Urschel et al.,1968; Li, 1987; Finkelstein et al., 1985; Kelly et al., 1992; Maruyama et al., 1993). In hypertension, the arteries are stiffer with reduced compliance and increased peripheral resistance (Mulvany, 1984; Folkow, 1990; Berger and Li, 1990), which increases the external work of the heart. The heart and the arterial system are coupled whether in acute hypertension (Berger and Li, 1992) or chronic hypertension (Roman et al., 1992). To unload the heart, pharmacological interventions are common (Frolich, 1985; Asmar et al., 1988; Perret et al., 1991). Vasodilators and β-adrenergic blockers are such examples (Grover et al., 1987; Zakzewski and Li, 1991). They exert dissimilar cardioarterial effects. Vasodilators primarily unload the heart by reducing the peripheral resistance, and thus reducing the BP, at the same time increasing ventricular outflow and improving large vessel compliance. β-adrenergic blockers, on the other hand, primarily act to reduce the workload of the heart by decreasing cardiac contractility. The reduced external work of the heart is accompanied by a decrease in BP, through a reduction in peripheral resistance and an increase in large vessel compliance (Simon et al, 1979,1992).

Myocardial ischemia is produced as a result of a reduction in CBF, which is associated with a decreased $O_2$ supply to tissues of the myocardium. Myocardial $O_2$ consumption ($MVO_2$) is intimately linked to the amount of CBF:

$$MVO_2 = Q_{cor} O_{2a-v} \qquad (6\text{-}24)$$

or that myocardial $O_2$ consumption is the product of CBF and arteriovenous $O_2$ difference. $O_2$ supply/demand ratio is particularly and acutely important for the coronary circulation, because the heart's ability to perform external work, EW, is dependent on its ability to efficiently extract $O_2$. Cardiac efficiency, $e$, is therefore defined as:

$$e = (EW)/(MVO_2) \qquad (6\text{-}25)$$

This aspect is discussed in Subheading 7.4., Allometry. It has been shown that pressure overload is more costly in terms of $O_2$ consumption than volume overload (Li, 1982).

Ischemia are predominantly regional. Regional ventricular response to acute occlusion of a coronary artery is characterized by paradoxical systolic bulging in the ischemic zone (e.g., Tennant and Wiggers, 1935; Theroux et al., 1977; Li, 1987; Drzewiecki et al., 1997). In assessing regional ventricular function, investigators have tackled the problem from a geometric perspective. Longitudinally, occlusion of a coronary artery produces normal and ischemic zones (Braunwald et al., 1976; Li, 1987,1993). Differential mechanical responses of myocardial layers and zones, defined by ischemia have been documented by studies of segment muscle contraction, wall thickness, and CBF measurements in these regions. Transversely, ischemia affect differentially the subepicardial and the subendocardial layers of the myocardium (Weintraub et al., 1981). Transmural wall-thickness changes have also been observed (Sasayama et al., 1981). These studies reported segmental lengthening, thinning of the myocardium (Gallagher et al., 1987) and reduced $MVO_2$ in the ischemic zone, reduced shortening, wall thickness, and CBF in the border zone; and the utilization of the Frank-Starling mechanism (Lew et al., 1985; Li, 1987; Fig. 6-26) and increased systolic shortening and wall thickness in the normal zone. The complexity of the structure and function of the myocardium is apparent. This is particularly evident during myocardial ischemia (Fig. 6-25).

Globally speaking, the P-V loop represents the external mechanical work generated during ventricular ejection (Li, 1987). Regionally, tension– or pressure–length loops have been found useful in representing the mechanical performance of the local myocardium (Hood et al., 1969; Tyberg et al, 1974; Forrester et al, 1974; Li, 1993). With myocardial ischemia, the cardiac muscle segment shortening is substituted by passive lengthening and the effective segment work becomes negative. This is seen in Fig. 6-27, in which the pressure–segment loop area becomes narrower and displays a loop area that resembles a figure 8. With pressure overloading, such as descending thoracic aortic occlusion, an increase in ventricular pressure is necessary to provide additional work to overcome the load, although the effective shortening is reduced. With β-blockers, there is a parallel shift to the right, indicating reduced cardiac contractility. The reduced segment work is also seen, showing an unloading characteristic.

The interaction of the heart and the arterial system becomes more acute under diseased conditions. The occlusion of a CA induces myocardial ischemia. Chronic myocardial infarction results in decreased compliance of both the LV and the arterial system. Acute coronary occlusion can often induce pulsus alternans. Thus, the alternating strong and weak contraction

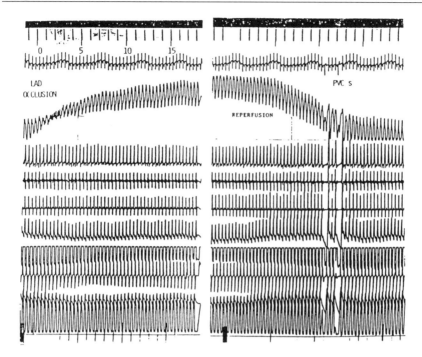

Fig. 6-25. Simultaneously measured hemodynamic parameters at the onset of the left anterior descending coronary artery (left), and during reperfusion (right) after 15 min of occlusion. Time marks are in seconds. Tracings from top. electrocardiogram (ECG), ischemic zone segment length ($L_1$), ascending aortic flow (Q), flow acceleration (dQ/dt), femoral arterial pressure derivative ($dP_{fem}/dt$), femoral arterial pressure ($P_{fem}$), amplified left ventricular end-diastolic pressure ($P_{ved}$), first derivative of LV pressure ($dP_v/dt$), AoP ($P_a$) and LV ($P_v$). Adapted with permission from Li (1987).

of the heart results in strong and weak AP pulses, as seen from Fig. 6-28. The occurrence of pulsus alternans has been observed in weakened heart, such as in heart failure. Its mechanism has been suggested to be more related to the alternation in cardiac contractility rather than the Frank-Starling mechanism (Li, 1982a). This is because the end-distolic cardiac muscle lengths remain constant during alternation; the cardiac muscle lengths at end-systole alternate.

For the interaction of the heart and the arterial system, emphasis has mostly been placed on the effect of peripheral resistance on compromised ventricular function. The pulsatile interaction of the LV and the systemic arterial system parameters (Geipel and Li, 1991; Li et al., 1995) during myocardial ischemia, however, have been investigated only to a limited extent.

From the preceding analysis, we see that ventricular performance can be significantly altered when the heart itself is adversely affected, and when

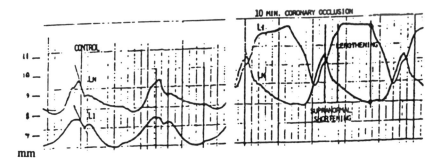

Fig. 6-26. Segment length recording of the normal and ischemic zones after ligation of the left anterior descending artery beyond first branching. Notice the passive lengthening in the ischemic zone and the supranormal shortening in the normal zone.

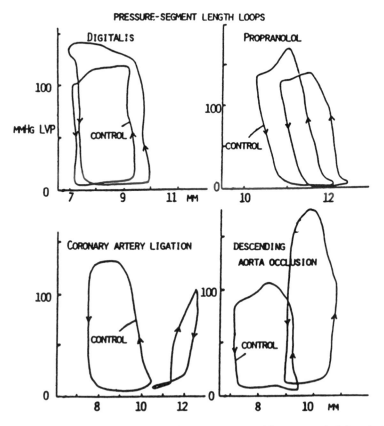

Fig. 6-27. LV pressure–segment length loops constructed from recorded signals during control and after coronary artery occlusion, during pressure-overloading by occlusion of descending thoracic aorta (DTA), and unloading with β-adrenergic blocker propranolol.

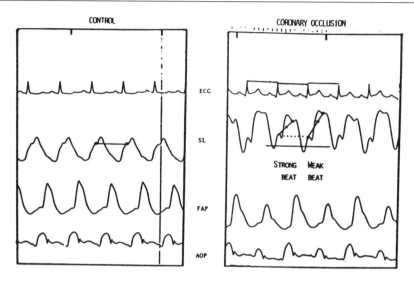

Fig. 6-28. Illustration of coronary artery occlusion induced pulsus alternans (right). End-diastolic lengths are constant (dotted line); end-systolic lengths alternate between strong and weak beats.

the ventricle encounters increased afterload, particularly during the ejection phase. The arterial system properties are therefore the major determinants under such circumstances. Arterial compliance ($C = dV/dP$) is a major determinant of the dynamic arterial load to the heart. Its use as a constant value throughout the cardiac cycle does not adequately characterize this load. Its pressure dependence signifies the importance of having an arterial system model that can realistically and accurately reflect the time-varying properties of the dynamic load. No previous investigators have proposed a model that incorporates this characteristic. We have devised a new arterial system model that incorporates a dynamic arterial compliance element that affords the computation of continuous variation of arterial compliance throughout the cardiac cycle ($C(P)$) (*see also* Chapters 3 and 7). Beat-to-beat compliance–pressure relation can be obtained (Li et al., 1986,1990; Li and Zhu, 1994). The temporal compliance–pressure relation provides a new means for investigating the dynamic behavior of the arterial system under pulsatile flow conditions (Li, 1998). A reduced arterial compliance impedes ventricular ejection flow and increases arterial pressure load, and signifies an alteration in cardiovascular structure and function. This provides a means to accurately quantify this dynamic load within each heartbeat during mechanically and vasoactively induced arterial hypertension (Li et al., 1994) and vasodilation (Li et al., 1996), as well as in myocardial ischemia.

We have concluded above that myocardial ischemia and hypertension have both been shown to be associated with a reduced arterial compliance, and are the major life-threatening cardiovascular diseases. Mortality is significantly increased when myocardial ischemia are present concurrently with arterial hypertension. Continuous variation of arterial compliance in a cardiac cycle is closely linked to ventricular ejection flow ($dV/dt$) and aortic distending pressure ($dP$). And, because ejection flow is determined by the amount of myocardial shortening, there must exist a relation between dynamic arterial compliance and cardiac muscle shortening. The mechanism giving rise to this relation is attributed to the active properties of the time-varying mechanical properties of the ventricle and the arterial system. Knowing the ventricular and arterial compliance variations within a cardiac cycle can, for example, provide a rapid method to effectively assess drug efficacy during routine catheterization or intraoperative procedures. This can be exercised by preferentially reversing the detrimental effects, which can favorably alter dynamic arterial compliance to improve myocardial shortening relation through active unloading the heart, as in the cases of hypertension and hypertension compounded myocardial ischemia.

# REFERENCES

Asmar, R. G., Pannier, B., Santoni, J., London, G. M., Levy, B. I., and Safar, M. E. Reversion of cardiac hypertrophy and reduced arterial compliance after converting enzyme inhibition in essential hypertension. *Circulation* 78:941–950, 1988.

Bellamy, R. F. and O'Benar, J. D. The determinants of the pressure-flow relation in the coronary vasculature. *J. Biomech. Eng.* 107:41–45, 1985.

Berger, D. S. and Li, J. K.-J. Temporal relationship between left ventricular and arterial system elastances. *IEEE Trans. Biomed. Eng.* 39:404–410, 1992.

Berger, D. S. and Li, J. K.-J. Concurrent compliance reduction and increased peripheral resistance in the manifestation of isolated systolic hypertension. *Am. J. Cardiol.* 65:67–71, 1990.

Berger, D. D., Lis, J. K.-J., and Noordergraaf, A. Arterial wave propagation phenomena, ventricular work, and power dissipation. *Ann. Biomed. Eng.* 23:804–811, 1995

Berne, R. M. and Levy, M. N. *Cardiovascular Physiology.* C.V. Mosby, St. Louis, 1986.

Beyar, R., Caminker, R., Manor, D. and Sideman, S. Coronary flow patterns in normal and ischemic hearts: transmyocardial and artery to vein distribution, *Ann. Biomed. Eng.* 21:435–458, 1993.

Braunwald, E., Ross, Jr., J., and Sonnenblick, E. H. *Mechanisms of Contradiction of the Normal and Failing Heart.* Little Brown, Boston, pp.357–397, 1976.

Bruinsma, P., Arts, T., Dankelman, J., and Spaan, J. A. E. Model of the coronary resistance and compliance, *Basic Res. Cardiol.* 83:510–524, 1988.

Canty, J. M., Jr., Klock, F. J., and Mates, R. E. Pressure and tone dependence of coronary diastolic input impedance and capacitance. *Am. J. Physiol.* 248:H700–711,1985.

Chilian, W. M. and Marcus, M. L. Coronary venous outflow persists after cessation of coronary arterial inflow. *Am. J. Physiol.* 247:H984–H990,1984.

Dai, J. and Li, J. K.-J. Prediction of impediment effect of cardiac contraction on coronary blood flow. *FASEB J.* 13:A424, 1999.

Dankelman, J., Spaan, J. A. E., Stassen, H. G., and Vergroesen, I. Dynamics of coronary adjustment to a change in heart rate in the anaesthetized goat, *J. Physiol.* 408:295–312, 1989.

Dankelman, J., Spaan, J. A. E., Van der Ploeg, C. P. B., and Vergroesen, I . Dynamic response of the coronary circulation to a rapid change in its perfusion in the anesthetized goat, *J. Physiol.* 410:703–715, 1989.

Dart, A., Silagy, C., Dewar, E., Jennings, G., and McNeil, J. Aortic distensibility and left ventricular structure and function in isolated systolic hypertension. *Eur. Heart J.* 14:1465–1470, 1993.

De Bruyne, B. and Pijls, N. H. J. Coronary pressure measurements. *Primary Cardiol.* 21:28–32, 1995.

De Bruyne, B., et al. Intracoronary pressure measurements with a 0.015-inch fluid filled angioplasty guide wire. In: Serruys, P. W., Foley, D. P., and de Feyter, P. J., eds., *Quantitative Coronary Angiographiy in Clinical Practice*, Kluwer Academic, Norwell, MA, pp. 147–165, 1994.

De Tombe P. P., Jones, S., Burkhoff, D., Hunter, W. C., and Kass, D. Ventricular stroke work and efficiency both remain nearly optimal despite altered vascular loading. *Am. J. Physiol.* 264:H1817–H1824, 1993.

Di Mario, C., Krams, R., Gil, R., and Serruys, P. W. Slope of the instantaneous hyperemic diastolic coronary flow velocity-pressure relation: a new index for assessment of the physiological significance of coronary stenosis in humans. *Circulation* 90:1215–1224, 1994.

Doucette, J. W., Goto, M., Flynn, A. E., Austin, R. E., Jr., Husseini, W., and Hoffman, J. I. E. Effect of cardiac contraction and cavity pressure on myocardial blood flow. *Am. J. Physiol.* 265:H1342–H1352, 1993.

Downey, J. M. and Kirk, E. S. Inhibition of coronary flow by intra-vascular waterfall mechanism. *Circ. Res.* 36:753–760, 1975.

Drzewiecki, G., Field, S., Mubarak, I., and Li, J. K.-J. Effect of vascular growth pattern on lumen area and compliance using a novel pressure-area model for collapsible wessels. *Am. J. Physiol. (Heart Circ. Physiol.)* 273:H2030–2043, 1997.

Elzinga, E. and Westerhof, N. Pressure and flow generated by the left ventricle against different impedances. *Circ. Res.* 32:178–186, 1973.

Eng, C., Jentzer, J. H., and Kirk, E. S. Effects of the coronary capacitance on the interpretation of diastolic pressure-flow relationships. *Circ. Res.* 50:334–341, 1982.

Finkelstein, S. M., Cohn, J. N., Carlyle, P. F., and Carlyle, W. J. Vascular compliance in congestive heart failure. *Proc. 7th IEEE Conf. Eng. Med. Biol. Soc.*, 7:550–553, 1985.

Fitchett, D. H. LV-arterial coupling: interactive model to predict effect of wave reflections on LV energetics. *Am. J. Physiol.* 261:H1026–H1033, 1991.

Folkow, B. Structural factor in primary and secondary hypertension. *Hypertension* 16:89–101, 1990.

Forrester, J. S., Tyberg, J. V., Wyatt, H. L., Goldner, S., and Parmely, W. W. Pressure-length loop: a new method for simultaneous measurement of segmental and total cardiac function. *J. Appl. Physiol.* 37:711–775, 1974.

Franklin, S. S. and Weber, M. A. Measuring hypertensive cardiovascular risk: the vascular overload concept. *Am. Heart J.* 128:793–803, 1994.

Franklin S. S., Gustin IV, W., Wong, N. D., Larson, M. G., Weber, M. A., Kannel, W. B., and Levy, D. Hemodynamic patterns of age-related changes in blood pressure. The Framingham heart study. *Circ.* 96:308–315, 1997.

Frasch H., Kresh, J. Y., and Noordergraaf, A. Interpretation of coronary vascular perfuison. In: G. Drzewiecki, G. and Li, J. K.-J., eds., *Analysis and Assessment of Cardiovascular Function.* Springer-Verlag, New York, pp. 109–127, 1998.

Frolich, E. D. Antihypertensive therapy: new concepts and agents. *Cardiology* 72:349-365, 1985.

Gallagher, K. P., Gerren, R. A., Buda, A. J., and Dunham, W. R. Nonischemic dysfunction at the lateral margins of ischemic myocardium. In: Sideman, S. and Beyar, R., eds., *Activation, Metabolism, and Perfusion of the Heart.* Martinus Nijohff, New York, pp. 479–500, 1987.

Geipel, P. S. and Li, J. K.-J. Pulsatile interaction of the left ventricle and arterial system in myocardial ischemia. *Proc. 13th Int. Conf. Eng. Med. Biol.*, 13:2049-2050, 1991.

Goto, M., VanBavel, E., Giezeman, M. J., and Spaan, J. A. Vasodilatory effect of pulsatile pressure on coronary resistance vessels. *Circ. Res.* 79(5):1039–1045, 1996.

Gould, K. L., Lipscomb, K., and Hamilton, G. W. Physiologic basis for assessing critical coronary stenosis. Instantaneous flow response and regional distribution during coronary hyperemia as measures of coronary flow reserve. *Am. J. Cardiol.* 33(1):87–94, 1974.

Grover, G. J., Weiss, H. R., Kostis, J. B., Li, J. K.-J., Kovacs, T., and Kedem, J. Beta-adrenoceptor simulation and blockade during myocardial ischemia in dogs: effect on cardiac $O_2$ supply and consumption. *Eur. J. Pharmacol.* 142:103–113, 1987.

Hayoz, D., Tardy, Y., Perret, F., Waeber, B., Meister, J.-J., and Brunner, H. R. Noninvasive determination of arterial diameter and distensibility by echo-tracking techniques in hypertension. *J. Hypertension* 10(Suppl 5):95–100, 1992.

Hayashida, K., Sunakawa, K., Noma, M., Sugimachi, M., Ando, H., and Nakamura, M. Mechanical matching of the left ventricle with the arterial system in exercising dogs. *Circ. Res.* 71:481–489, 1992.

Hettrick, D. A. and Warltier, D. C. Ventriculoarterial coupling. In: Warltier, D. C., ed.,*Ventricular Function*, Wiliams & Wilkins, Baltimore, pp. 153–179, 1995.

Holensterin, R. and Nerem, R. M. Parameteric analyisi of flow in the intramyocardial circualtion. *Ann. Biomed. Eng.* 18:347–365, 1990.

Hoffman, J. I. Maximal coronary flow and the concept of coronary vascular reserve. *Circulation* 70:153–159, 1984.

Hoffman, J. I. E. and Spaan, J. A.E. Pressure-flow relations in coronary circulation. *Physiol. Rev.* 70:331–390, 1990.

Hood, W. B., Covelli, V. H., Abelman, W. H., and Normal, J. C. Persistence of contractile behavior in acutely ischemic myocardium. *Cardiovasc. Res.* 3:249–255, 1969.

Kelly, R. and Fitchett, D. Noninvasive determination of aortic input impedance and external left ventricular power output: a validation and repeatability study of a new technique. *J. Am. Coll. Cardiol.* 20:952–963, 1992.

Kelly, R. P., Tunin, R., Kass, D. A. Effect of reduced aortic compliance on cardiac efficiency and contractile function of in situ canine left ventricle. *Circ. Res.* 71:490–502, 1992.

Kelly, R. P., Ting, C.-T., Yang, T. M., Liu, C.-P., Maughan, W. L., Chang, M.-S., and Kass, D. A. Effective arterial elastance as index of arterial vascular load in humans. *Circulation* 86:513–521, 1992a.

Klocke, F. J. Measurements of coronary flow reserve: defining pathophysiology versus making decisions about patient care. *Circulation* 76:1183–1189, 1987.

Klocke, F. J., Mates, R. E., Canty, J. M., and Ellis, A. K. Coronary pressure-flow relationships: controversial issues and probable implications, *Circ. Res.* 56:310-323, 1985.

Krams, R., Sipkema, P., and Westerhof, N. Contractility is the main determinant of coronary systolic flow impediment. *Am. J. Physiol.* 257:H1936–H1944, 1989b.

Krams, R., Sipkema, P. and Westerhof, N. The varying elastance concept may explain coronary systolic flow impediment. *Am. J. Physiol.* 257:H1471–1479, 1989c.

Krayenbuhl, H. P., Hess, O. M., and Turina, J. Assessment of left ventricular function. *Cardiovasc. Med.* 3:883–910, 1978.

Lew, W. Y. and Ban-Hayashi, E. Mechanisms of improving regional and global ventricular function by preload alterations during acute ischemia in the canine left ventricle. *Circulation* 72:1125–1134, 1985.

Li, J. K.-J. Oxygen cost to work ratio in pressure-loaded ventricle. *Proc. 35th Ann. Conf. Eng. Med. Biol.* 24:145, 1982.

Li, J. K.-J. Ventricualr alternans: relative unimportance of the Starling mechanism. *IRCS J. Med. Sci.* 10:19–20, 1982a.

Li, J. K.-J. and Zhu, Y. Arterial compliance and its pressure dependence in hypertension and vasodilation. *Angiology, J. Vasc. Dis.* 45:113–117, 1994.

Li, J. K.-J. *Arterial System Dynamics.* New York University Press, New York, 1987.

Li, J. K.-J., Cui, T., and Drzewieki, G. Nonliniar model of the arterial system incorporating a pressure-dependent compliance. *IEEE Trans. Biomed. Eng.* BME-37:673–678, 1990.

Li, J. K.-J., Drzewiecki, G., and Wang, R. P. Compliance of the aorta during acute pressure loading. *Proc. 7th Int. Conf. Cardiovasc. Syst. Dynamics*, 7:1–3, 1986.

Li, J. K.-J., Zhu, Y., Wang, J.-J., and Drzewiecki, G. Sensitivity of measured and model-derived parameters for assessing myocardial ischemia and hypertension. *Ann. Biomed. Eng.* 23:S38, 1995

Li, J. K.-J., Zhu, Y., and Drzewieck, G. Arterial compliance changes in spontaneous hypertension and hypotension. *FASEB J.* A462, 1993a.

Li, J. K.-J., Zhu, Y., and Drzewieck, G. Difference in arterial compliance values measured at systolic, mean and diastolic blood pressure. *Am. J. Hypertension*, 6:41A, 1993b.

Li, J. K.-J., Zhu, Y., and Drzewiecki, G. Pulse pressure is a significant determinant of arterial compliance in hypertension and vasodilation. *Circulation* 90:I166, 1994.

Li, J. K.-J. Feedback effects in heart-arterial system interaction. *Adv. Exp. Med. Biol.* 346:325–333, 1993.

Li, J. K.-J. Regional ventricular function in myocardial ischemia. In: Sideman, S. and Beyar, R., eds., *Activation, Metabolism and Perfusion of the Heart.* Martinus Nijhoff, pp. 453–461, 1987.

Li, J. K.-J., Zhu, Y., and Drzewiecki, G. Systemic arterial compliance dependence on blood pressure: global effects. *J. Cardiovasc. Diagn. Proc.* 13:300, 1996.

Li, J. K.-J. A new description of arterial function: the compliance-pressure loop. *Angiology, J. Vasc. Dis.* 49:543–548, 1998.

Little, W. C. and Cheng, C.-P. Left ventricular-arterial coupling in conscious dogs. *Am. J. Physiol.* 261:H70–76, 1991.

Marcus M.L. *Coronary Circulation in Health and Disease.* McGraw-Hill, New York, 1983.

Maruyama, Y., Nishioka, O., Nozaki, E., Kinoshita, H., Kyono, H., Koiwa, Y., and Takishima, T. Effects of arterial distensibility on left ventricular ejection in the depressed contractile state. *Cardiovasc. Res.* 27:182–187, 1993.

Mates, R. E. and Judd, R. M. Models of coronary pressure-flow relations. *Adv. Exp. Med. Biol.* 346:153–161, 1993.

Mates, R. E. Coronary capacitance. *Prog. Cardiovasc. Dis.* 31:1–15, 1988.

Maughan, W. L., Sunagawa, K., Burkoff, D., and Sagawa, K. Effect of arterial impedance changes on the end-systolic pressure-volume realtion. *Circ. Res.* 54:595–602, 1984.

Meister, J.-J., Tardy, Y., Stergiopulos, N., Hayoz, D., Brunner, H. R., and Etienne, J.-D. Non-invasive method for the assessment of non-linear elastic properties and stress of forearm arteries in vivo. *J. Hypertension* 10(S6):23–26, 1992.

Mulvany, M. J. Determinants of vascular hemodynamic characteristics. *Hypertension* 6(Suppl. III):13–18, 1984.

Nichols, W. W., O'Rourke, M. F., Avolio, A. P., Yaginuma, T., Murgo, J. P., Pepine, C. J., and Conti, C. R. Effects of age on ventricular vascular coupling. *Am. J. Cardiol.* 55:1179–1184, 1985.

Olsson, R. A., Bunger, R. and Spaan, J. A. E. Coronary circulation. In: Fozzard, H. A., Haber, E., Jennings, R. B., Katz, A. M., and Morgan, H. E., eds., *The Heart and Cardiovascular System*, 2nd ed., Raven Press, New York, pp. 1393–1425, 1992.

O'Rourke, M. F. Arterial hemodynamics in hypertension. *Circ. Res.* 26(Suppl. II):123–132, 1970.

Perret, F., Mooser, V., Hayoz, D., Tardy, Y., Meister, J.-J., Etienne, J.-D., et al. Evaluation of arterial compliance pressure curves. Effects of antihypertensive drugs. *Hypertension* 18(Suppl. II):77–83, 1991.

Rabbany, S. Y., Kresh, J. Y., and Noordergraaf, A. Intramyocardial pressure: interatction of myocardial fluid pressure and fiber stress. *Am. J. Physiol.* 257:H357–H364 (1989).

Reneman, R. S. and Arts, T. Dynmaic capacitance of epicardial coronart arteries in vivo. *J. Biomech. Eng.* 107:29–33, 1985.

Roman, M. J., Saba, P. S., Pini, R., Spitzer, M., Pickering, T. G., et al. Parallel cardiac and vascular adaptation in hypertension. *Circulation* 86:1909–1918, 1992.

Safar, M. E., Simon, A. C., and Levenson, J. A. Structural changes of large arteries in sustained essential hypertension. *Hypertension*, 6(Suppl. III):117–121, 1984.

Sasayama, S., Gallagher, K. P., Kemper, W. S., Franklin, D., and Ross, J., Jr. Regional left ventricular wall thickness early and late after coronary occlusion in the conscious dog. *Am. J. Physiol.* 240:H293–299, 1981.

Segal, J., Kern, M. J., Scott, N. A., et al. Alterations of phasic coronary artery flow velocity in humans during percutaneous angioplasty. *J. Am. Coll. Cardiol.* 20:276–286, 1992.

Sideman S. and Beyar, R. *Simulation and Modeling of the Cardiac System.* Matinus Nijhoff, New York, 1987.

Simon, A. C., Levenson, J., Chau, N. P., and Pithois-Merli, I. Role of arterial compliance in the physiopharmacological approach to human hypertension. *J. Cardiovasc. Pharmacol.* 19(S5):D11–S20, 1992.

Simon, A. C., Safar, M. E., Levenson, J. A., London, G. M., Levy, B. I., and Chau, N. P. Evaluation of large arteries compliance in man. *Am. J. Physiol.* 237:H550–554, 1979.

Spaan, J. A. E. Mechanical determinants of myocardial perfusion. *Basic Res. Cardiol.* 90:89–102, 1995.

Spaan, J. A. E. Intramyocardial compliance studies by venous outflow at arterial occlusion. *Circulation* 66(Suppl. 3):307, (Abstract), 1981a.

Spaan, J. A. E., Breuls, N. P. W.,and Laird, J. D. Diastolic-systolic coronary flow differences are caused by intramyocardial pump action in the anesthetized dog. *Circ. Res.* 49:584–593, 1981b.

Starling, M.R. Left ventricular-arterial coupling relations in the normal human heart. *Am. Heart J.* 125:1659–1666, 1993.

Suga, H., Igarashi, Y., Yamada, O., and Goto, Y. Mechanical efficiency of the left ventricle as a function of preload, afterload and contractility. *Heart Vessels* 1:3–8, 1985.

Suga, H., Sagawa, K., and Shoukas, A. Load independence of the instantaneous pressure-volume ratio of the canine left ventricle and effects of epinephrine and heart rate on the ratio. *Circ. Res.* 32:314–322, 1973.

Sunagawa, K., Maughan, W. L., Burkhoff, D., Sagawa, K. Left ventricular interaction with arterial load studied in isolated canine left ventricle. *Am. J. Physiol.* 265:H773–780, 1983.

Sunagawa, K., Maughan, W. L., and Sagawa, K. Optimal arterial resistance for the maximal stroke work studied in isolated canine left ventricle. *Circ. Res.* 56:586–585, 1985.

Tennant, R. and Wiggers, C. J., Effect of coronart occlusion on myocardial contraction. *Am. J. Physiol.* 112:351–361, 1935.

Theroux, P., Ross, J., Jr., Franklin, D., Covell, J. W., Bloor, C. M., and Sasayama, S. Regional myocardial function and dimensions early and late after myocardial infarction in the unanesthetized dog. *Circ Res* 40: 158-165, 1977.

Tyberg, J. V., Forrester, J. S., Wyatte, H. L., Goldner, S. J., Parmley., W. W., and Swan, H. J. C. An analysis of segment ischemic dysfunction utilizing the pressure-length loop. *Circulation* 49:748–747, 1974.

Urschel, C. W., Corell, J. W., Sonnenblick,E. H., Ross, J., Jr., and Braunwald, E. Effects of decreased aortic compliance on performance of the left ventricle. *Am. J. Physiol.* 214:298–304, 1968.

Van den Horn, G. J., Westerhof, N.,and Elzinga, G. Interaction of heart and arterial system. *Ann. Biomed. Eng.* 12:151–162, 1984.

Van Huis, G. A., Sipkema, P., and Westerhof, N. Coronary input impedance during the cardiac cycle as determined by impulse response method. *Am. J. Physiol.* 253:H317–H324 (1987),

Vis, M. A., Bovendeerd, P. H. M., Sipkema, P., and Westerhof, N. Effect of ventricular contraction, pressure, and wall stretch on vessels at different locations in the wall. *Am. J. Physiol.* 272:H2963–2975 (1997),

Vis, M. A., Spikema, P., and Westerhof, N. Modeling pressure-area relations of coronary blood vessels embedded in cardiac muscle in diastole and systole. *Am. J. Physiol.* 268:H2531–H2543 (1995),

Weintraub, W. S., Hattori, S., Agarwal, J. B., Bodenheimer, M. M., Banka, V. S., and Helfant, R. H. Relationship between myocardial blood flow and contraction by myocardial layer in the canine left ventricle during ischemia. *Circ. Res.* 48:430–438, 1981.

Zhu, Y., Li, J. K.-J., and Drzewieck, G. Arterial compliance variation throughout the cardiac cycle. *Proc. IEEE 14th Int. Conf. Eng. Med. Biol.* pp. 758–759, 1992a.

Zhu, Y., et al, Arterial wave reflections and left ventricular energy output in vasoconstriction and vasodilation. *Proc. 18th NE Bioeng. Conf.*, pp. 125–126, 1992b.

Zinemanas, D., Beyar, R., and Sideman, S. Intramyocardial fluid transport effects on coronary flow and LV mechanics. In: Sideman, S. and Beyarm R., eds., *Interactive Phenomena in the Cardiac System*, Plenum, New York, pp. 219–231, 1993.

# 7 New Approaches to Clinical Evaluations

## 7.1. Hypertension, Vascular Stiffness, and Arterial Compliance

### 7.1.1. HEMODYNAMICS OF HYPERTENSION

The necessity of the transmission of pressure and flow pulses, in order to perfuse organ vascular beds, puts a burden on the arterial conduits. The pulsation associated with each heartbeat presents periodical variations in blood pressure (BP). The pulse pressure (PP) exerted on the blood vessel wall manifests itself as cyclic stress on the wall. The greater the PP at any given mean pressure level, the greater the cyclic stress (Fig. 7-1). Cyclic stress has been shown to induce material fatigue. The consequence is the derangement of normal organization of blood vessel wall structures. At higher mean pressure levels, increased pulse becomes more threatening to mechanical function of the arteries, as well as to the heart. Increased mean pressure increases vascular resistance; increased PP is associated with increased vascular stiffness and decreased blood vessel compliance. This is easily seen from simultaneous recording of aortic pressure (AoP) and pulsatile diameter at normal and high BP conditions (Fig. 7-2). With increased BP, the vessel distends to a larger diameter, but the proportional change in diameter ($\Delta D$), with respect to its mean value (D), or radial strain, is greatly reduced. Vascular changes in hypertension differ among the aorta, large and small arterie,s and arterioles. Vascular growth and hypertrophy have also been observed (Drzewiecki et al., 1997).

There are several forms of hypertension (e.g., Pickering, 1972). The most common form is known as essential hypertension, the origins of which are still unclear. The hemodynamic aspects will be dealt here. The conventional definition of human hypertension in terms of BP levels is based on the systolic and diastolic blood pressures (SBP and DBP) measured from the brachial artery. This has generally been defined as a SBP over 140 mmHg and a DBP over 90 mmHg. The range between 140/90 and the normal SBP/DBP pressure of 120/80 has been defined as borderline hypertension. However, it should be recognized that brachial arterial systolic pressure is normally greater and diastolic pressure smaller than central AoP, as shown in Chapter 4.

From: *Arterial Circulation: Physical Principles and Clinical Applications*
By: J. K-J. Li © Humana Press Inc., Totowa, NJ

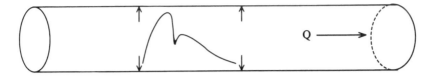

Fig. 7-1. Chronic cyclic stress sustained by the viscoelastic arterial lumen under variable PP amplitude.

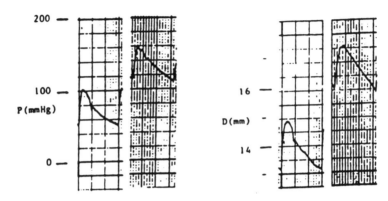

Fig. 7-2. Simultaneously recorded AoP and ultrasonic diameter under normal and high BP conditions in dog aorta. Despite the increase in mean diameter, the pulsatile change in diameter is reduced in hypertension.

Hypertension reflects the increased tension on the blood vessel wall. It has been long known that arterial hypertension is associated with an increased peripheral resistance (PR) (e.g., Pickering, 1936,1955). The concurrent reduction in arterial compliance has also been reported (Li et al., 1986; Simon et al., 1979,1992; Randall et al., 1984; Safar et al., 1984; Asmar et al., 1988; Berger and Li, 1990). Alterations in compliance and resistance reflect changes in the mechanical properties of the vessel walls and the state of the perfusing vascular beds (Li, 1987,1996). Successful antihypertensive therapy must be able to normalize both vascular resistance and compliance to normal levels, to have any long-term impact or adequate vascular remodeling to return BP to normal levels.

Regarding cardiac function, left ventricular (LV) outflow is dependent on its systemic arterial load. Arterial compliance and peripheral vascular resistance comprise the major components of this load. Peripheral resistance is associated with steady flow; arterial compliance is associated with dynamic changes, and hence, pulsatile pressure–flow behavior. Both reduced arterial compliance and increased peripheral resistance impede ventricular outflow (Fig. 7-3), as seen in the previous chapter. There is a

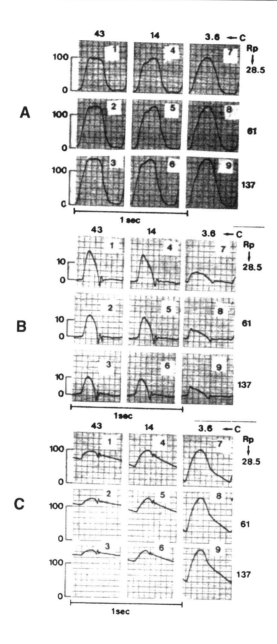

Fig. 7-3. (**A**) LV pressure, (**B**) ventricular ejection flow, and (**C**) AoP facing different levels of arterial compliance and peripheral resistance. Increased resistance and reduced compliance both serve to decrease ventricular ejection (B9) and increase PP (C9). Adapted with permission from Elzinga and Westerhof (1973).

close relationship between arterial structure and function and overall cardiac function and structure, e.g., increased arterial pressure has been shown to reduce myocardial shortening (Li, 1987; Zhu, 1996; *also see* Chapter 6). Roman et al. (1992,1996) found that concentric left ventricular hypertrophy (LVH) is associated with increased carotid arterial wall thickness, cross-sectional area, and elastic modulus. They followed the method by Ilercil et al. (1995), with simultaneous noninvasive recording of the carotid pulse and vessel diameter by M-mode ultrasound echocardiograph. Chronic pressure-overload, such as hypertension, generally induces concentric hypertrophy. Increased LV mass (Frolich et al., 1985,1992; Devereux and Roman, 1993) and its reversal with antihypertension drugs have attracted clinical interests.

The fact that, in some hypertension cases, the stroke volume (SV) remain unchanged, suggests a role of cardiac origin in hypertension. Sympathetic overstimulation and increased cardiac contractility can both augment SBP. The exact mechanisms by which these two factors come about have not been made clear.

In hypertension, the arteries are stiffer, with reduced compliance and increased peripheral resistance. This increases the external work of the heart, through increased pulse wave velocity (PWV) (Li et al., 1996) and increased wave reflections because of impedance mismatching (Li et al., 1984; Li, 1989). Pharmacological treatment to reduce BP and unload the heart (Simon et al., 1992; Opie, 1995) through β-adrenergic blockers (Corbo et al., 1989), vasodilators (Kelly et al., 1990; Li and Zhu, 1994), diuretics (Levenson et al., 1992), and angiotensin-converting enzyme inhibitors (Zakzewski et al., 1992; Ting et al., 1993), are common, because the heart and the arterial system are closely coupled (Li, 1993,1996; Trazzi et al., 1993; Roman et al., 1996). We have shown in Chapter 6 that the time-varying compliance of the LV exhibits a close relation to pressure-dependent arterial system compliance (Berger and Li, 1992). Both the maximum elastance of the left ventricle ($E_{max}$) and the maximum elastance (inverse of compliance) of the arterial system occur at end-systole. The study of the pressure-dependent behavior of arterial compliance or vascular stiffness is important, because of its relevance to many cardiovascular diseases, particularly hypertension and atherosclerosis, which are results of alterations in the mechanical properties of the vessel wall and the vascular states. In hypertension, for instance, the increased pressure is always associated with a reduced arterial compliance. A decreased compliance can occur as a consequence of an elevated AP, which may in turn be related to decreased compliance as a result of alterations in vessel wall properties. The compliance–pressure loop shown in Subheading 7.1.3.4. can be used to separate arterial wall properties from the pressure–flow effects.

The compliance–pressure curve has been given by some investigators for individual arteries, such as the human radial and brachial arteries (Trazzi et al., 1993; Meister et al., 1992). In these arteries, arterial compliance was found to also exhibit an inverse exponential relation to pressure, as given in Eq. 7-5. These, as well as other investigators, did not demonstrate the continuous change of arterial compliance as a function of pressure for the entire cardiac cycle. However, they did show that a larger artery has a larger compliance and a greater dependence on pressure, and that arterial compliance is reduced in hypertension, as expected.

The pressure–strain elastic modulus (Chapter 2) is a popular clinical means to assess blood vessel compliance or distensibility. $Ep$ is calculated from the measurement of the pulsatile arterial distending pressure, $\Delta p$, and the corresponding pulsatile change in vessel diameter, $\Delta D$, in relation to mean diameter, $D$. This approach can be accomplished by noninvasive ultrasound and plethysmograph assessment of compliance and distensibility of blood vessels (Meister et al., 1992; Milio et al., 1997).

### 7.1.2. Vascular Impedance in Hypertension

Apart from those values and contour changes observed in MP, researchers have long focused on the structural and hemodynamic changes in the arterial system contributing to the alteration in MP.

Despite of the complex wave phenomena in the arterial tree, the input impedance offers a relatively simple form to describe structural changes. The modified three-element windkessel model, as described in Chapter 3, lumps the features of the arterial system into three main hemodynamic parameters, namely, the total peripheral resistance ($Rs$), total arterial compliance ($C$), and characteristic impedance ($Z_o$) of the proximal aorta. Compliance is the ratio of the changes in volume ($dV$) resulting from a change in transmural distending pressure ($dP$) or $dV/dP$. This is defined by the slope of the pressure–volume (P-V) relationship. The characteristic impedance depends only on the mechanical and geometric properties of the aorta. $Z_o$ represents the proximal central aorta and $Rs$ represents the peripheral vascular contribution, and the compliance represents the contributions from the distributing arteries. Large arteries contribute greater amounts to the total arterial compliance, mostly because of their greater distensibility and large lumen volumes.

The effects of altered total peripheral resistance and compliance on pressure pulse contour have been shown by Li and Berger (1989) and Berger and Li (1990). An increased resistance leads to an increase in mean blood pressure. Under this condition, when arterial distensibility is not altered, systolic and diastolic pressure are both increased by an equal proportion. Arterial distensibility is related to pulsatile pressure, it damps the pulsatility of pressure: The lower the arterial compliance, the higher the pulsatility of systemic BP. A decrease in arterial compliance alone without change in peripheral resistance results in an increase in systolic pressure and a decrease in diastolic pressure. If this occurs with a concurrent increase in $R_s$, mean pressure is then significantly increased and accompanied with a much greater rise in systolic pressure and a lesser rise in diastolic pressure.

Total peripheral resistance is determined by the viscous properties of blood and vessel caliber, its increment in hypertension is usually the result of an increase in arteriolar tone and/or decrease total vascularity of tissue and it determines the relationship between mean blood pressure and mean flow. Because the heart pumps intermittently, resistance, by itself, cannot describe the overall load presented to the heart. The input impedance of the arterial system, expressed in the modified windkessel model, gives a closer description of the system, both for steady and oscillatory components of pressure and flow waveform. Significant increases in magnitude and oscillations in input impedance have been found in hypertension. This includes an increase in overall peripheral resistance (zero frequency component), and increase in characteristic impedance (Merillon et al., 1982). The impedance minimum is shifted generally to the right, with increased frequency of the first minimum. Fluctuation in modulus and phase of impedance is caused by wave reflection at peripheral sites (O'Rourke and Taylor, 1966), the frequencies at which the fluctuations occur depend on the distance and wave velocity between heart and reflection site. It can be concluded that elevated BPs are attributed to earlier return of reflected wave because of increase in wave velocity.

Both input impedance and characteristic impedance moduli increase as the measurement site becomes farther away from the heart. Because compliance resides mosty in the aorta, the proximal vessels contribute greatly to the capacitive load, and periphery contributes to the resistive load. The number of frequency-dependent reflections dominates the change. The reflection is large and variable, because of the periphery at low frequencies; it is small and constant at high frequencies, because of proximal vessels. The mean pressure to mean flow ratio is significantly higher than oscillating components (PP and flow). Therefore, the heart appears to be decoupled from its peripheral load at high frequencies.

### 7.1.3. ARTERIAL COMPLIANCE IN HYPERTENSION

In Chapter 2, the P-V relations in arteries are shown to be curvilinear, i.e., arteries stiffen when pressurized, so that a greater distending pressure is necessary to dilate the arterial lumen to allow pulsatile volume of blood to be transmitted from one segment to the next. This increased stiffness is related to the structure of the arterial wall, which implies that the compli-

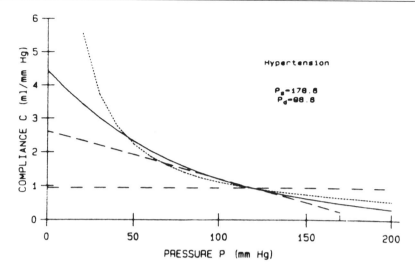

Fig. 7-4. Compliance vs pressure for a hypertensive patient. Compliance decreases with increasing pressure, but the windkessel model predicted compliance shows a constant value. Adapted with permission from Liu et al. (1986).

ance-pressure relation is not a constant one. Indeed, arterial compliance has been found to be smaller at higher pressures. Figure 7-4 illustrates the decreased compliance with increasing BP in a hypertensive patient (Liu et al. 1986; Ting et al., 1993). This pressure-dependence is not seen if compliance is calculated from the linear windkessel model, which gives a constant compliance at all pressure levels.

In hypertension, ventricular ejected volume, or stroke volume is normally maintained at the expense of a greatly increased arterial pressure load, which results in increased cardiac work and myocardial oxygen consumption. The reduced arterial compliance associated with hypertension has been shown to increase PP, and consequently the oscillatory component of external cardiac work. This increase in PP is related to an increased arterial stiffness, which also manifests in an increase in PWV. Hence, change in arterial compliance has been used as a compass of arterial wall behavior, as well as an effective parameter for assessing therapeutic treatment efficacy.

The effects on BP because of changes in arterial compliance and peripheral resistance are well known. An increase in $R_s$ results in an increased mean pressure, and, if $C$ is unchanged, systolic and diastolic pressure would both increase. Changing $C$ should have no effect on mean pressure, if the flow waveform remains unchanged. A decrease in $C$ would result in an increased systolic pressure and a decreased diastolic pressure. Specifically, the effect of decreasing $C$ and increasing $R_s$ would result in a combined and a larger increase in $P_s$ than $P_d$. Changing compliance can alter the arrival of wave reflections, and can significantly alter SBP (Li et al., 1996b). There are four general approaches to the assessment of arterial compliance. These are defined below.

### 7.1.3.1. Stroke Volume to Pulse Pressure Ratio in Hypertension

$$C_v = SV/PP \tag{7-1}$$

This formula may overestimate compliance, because SV is used to represent dV, which may also include the effect of LV compliance. This provides the systolic index of arterial compliance, since both SV and PP are determined in systole.

Recently, De Simone et al. (1992,1995,1999) showed that the survival rate for patients with reduced SV/PP ratio is considerably less than those with higher SV/PP ratio, when age and LV mass are taken into account (Fig. 7-5). The revival of this simple index of arterial compliance has received considerable interest.

### 7.1.3.2. Diastolic Pressure Decay Time Constant.

$$\tau = \frac{t_d}{\ln(P_{ed}/P_d)} \tag{7-2}$$

and

$$C_\tau = \frac{t_d}{R_s \ln (P_{ed}/P_d)} \tag{7-3}$$

This is shown in Chapter 3, and is derivable from the windkessel model. This provides the diastolic index of arterial compliance, since only the diastolic aortic pressure is used in determining the decay time constant, $\tau$.

### 7.1.3.3. Arterial Compliance Calculated From Vascular Impedance.

At low frequencies, vascular impedance has a negative phase, which primarily results from the capacitive effect, hence compliance. Arterial compliance can be obtained from the following relation:

$$C_\omega = \frac{1}{\omega|Z|} \tag{7-4}$$

This represents the frequency domain method of the determination of arterial compliance, and is valid at low frequencies, when the phase of the input impedance is negative. Here Z is the magnitude of the impedance. Comparisons of total arterial system compliance derived from input impedance, diastolic aortic pressure decay, and the ratio of SV/PP have been given by Geipel and Li (1990) and Zhu et al. (1995a). Some of these results are shown in Fig. 7-6.

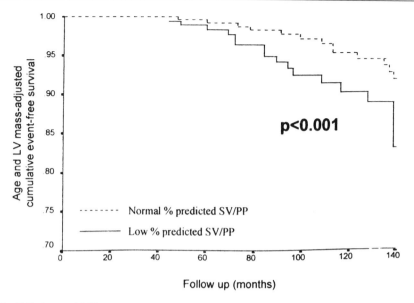

Fig. 7-5. Age and LV mass adjusted cumulative event-free survival graph as a function of follow-up. This graph shows reduced survival rate follows a reduced SV/PP. Adapted with permission from De Simone et al. (1999).

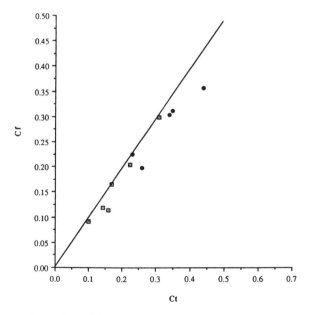

Fig. 7-6. Comparison of arterial system compliance calculated from the time domain from the diastolic AoP decay time constant, $C\tau$, and from the frequency domain from the low frequency modulus of input impedance, $C\omega$ or $C_f$.

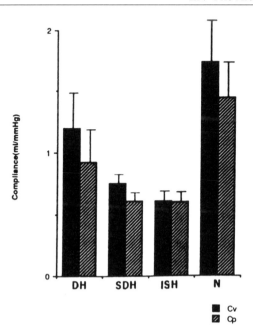

Fig. 7-7. Comparison of arterial compliances calculated from the diastolic AoP decay time constant ($C_\tau$ or $C_p$) and from the ratio of SV/PP ($C_v$) in four groups of subjects. N = normal adults, ISH = isolated systolic hypertension, DH = diastolic hypertension, SDH = elevated SBP and DBP.

Iantorno and Li (1988) have investigated changes in total arterial compliance in three different types of hypertension. Arterial compliance calculated from the diastolic aortic pressure decay time constant ($C_\tau$ or $C_p$) and the ratio of SV/PP ($C_v$) were compared in four groups of subjects. These are normal adults, isolated systolic hypertensives (ISHs), diastolic hypertensives (DHs), and hypertensives with both elevated systolic and diastolic blood pressure (SDHs). The results are summarized in Fig. 7-7. All hypertensives are seen to have reduced total arterial system compliance when compared to normal individuals. The decrease is small in DH, mostly because of lower PP and overall mean pressure. Patients with ISH and SDH exhibit significantly greater reduction in arterial compliance. In addition, it can be seen that either method of determining arterial compliance can differentiate the arterial compliance changes.

**7.1.3.4. Instantaneous or Pressure-Dependent Arterial Compliance Characteristics.** The pressure dependence of arterial compliance has been well recognized and is discussed in Chapters 2 and 3. This is seen from experimental observations, in which arteries stiffen when pressurized (Peterson, 1960) The decreased compliance with increasing BP is more pronounced in large vessels, such as the aorta. But this phenomenon has also been reported in other arteries in experimental animals (Cox,1975) and in humans. This increased stiffness is related to the structural component properties of the arterial walls. This also implies that the compliance–pressure relation is not a constant one (Li et al., 1993b), as suggested by the classical windkessel model of the arterial system. This popular model formulation assumes that the compliance of the arterial system remains constant throughout the cardiac cycle. Hence, compliance in systole and in diastole are assumed to be the same, despite varying pressure amplitudes (PP). We have shown that PP is a significant determinant of arterial compliance, even within a single cardiac cycle (Li et al., 1994).

The pressure dependence of arterial compliance has been known for some time, but, only recently, the pressure-dependent compliance characteristics of the arterial system could be quantified (Li et al., 1990) during hypertension and subsequent vasodilatation (Li and Zhu, 1994). Here, we introduce the compliance–pressure loop to demonstrate how total arterial compliance can be influenced by the vessel wall properties, as well as instantaneous pressure–flow relation.

Arterial compliance, either of a single vessel or of the whole arterial system, has been shown to be dependent on the level of BP in an inverse exponential relation (Li et al., 1990; Capello et al., 1995). This can be expressed as

$$C(P(t)) = a \exp [bP(t)] \tag{7-5}$$

where a and b are constants. The exponent b is normally negative. Thus, compliance is seen to decline exponentially with increasing pressure. This is illustrated in Fig. 7-8, in which the arterial compliance is plotted against mean pressure, the total arterial system compliance declines exponentially, following Eq. 7-5. The constant, a, is 1.024, and the exponent, b, is −0.0079, in this example. The characteristic impedance is also shown as a function of frequency. In general, it increases with increasing mean pressure. However, it constitutes a much weaker dependence on mean blood pressure within the range investigated.

This pressure-dependent compliance, $C(P)$, is used to substitute for the constant compliance, $C$, of the three-element windkessel model representation of the arterial system. This latter model also consists of the resistance of the peripheral vascular beds ($R_s$), and the characteristic impedance of the proximal aorta ($Z_o$). The following expression relates the measured AoP ($P_a$), aortic flow ($Q$), and characteristic impedance

$$P_a(t) = Q(t) Z_o + P(t) \tag{7-6}$$

Aortic flow obtained from animal experimental data was used as input. Initial values of a and b were first estimated based on curve-fitting of

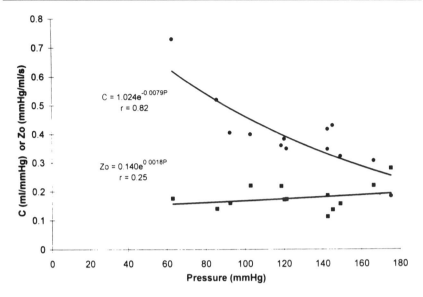

Fig. 7-8. Total arterial system compliance and characteristic impedance of dog aota plotted as a function of mean BP. Compliance declined exponentially with increasing pressure. Characteristic impedance increased slightly with increasing MP.

windkessel model compliance vs pressure data obtained for a number of beats. The initial value of $P$ was chosen as diastolic aortic pressure, $P_d$. This set of initial values were adjusted until the least-squares error, $E$, between measured and predicted AoP is minimized to meet the desired error within physiological limits,

$$E = \sum_{i=1}^{N} [P_a \text{ calculated } (t_i) - P_a \text{ measured } (t_i)]^2 \qquad (7\text{-}7)$$

where $N$ is the total number of sampled points within one complete cardiac cycle.

The temporal relation of arterial compliance and BP can be represented by the compliance-pressure loop. This loop can be constructed by plotting the pressure-dependent arterial compliance ($C(P)$) point-by-point against measured AoP ($P_a$) for one complete cardiac cycle.

In order to demonstrate the usefulness of the compliance–pressure loop, experimental data was obtained from spontaneous hypertension, which was induced by intravenous bolus infusion of a potent vasoconstrictor, methoxamine (2–5 mg/mL). This normally increased BP transiently to different high levels suitable for examination of acute hypertension conditions. The loops are obtained for each of the selected beats during control and acute hypertension conditions. As expected, hemodynamic data showed significantly increased BP and peripheral resistance during acute

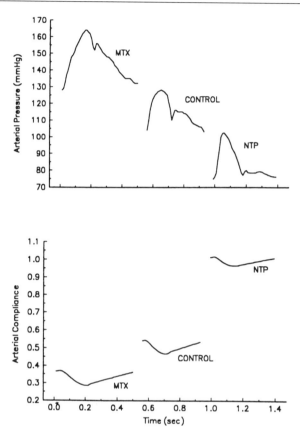

Fig. 7-9. Aortic blood pressue waveforms and the corresponding instantaneous pressure-dependent compliances obtained at control (center), methoxamine (MTX)-induced vasoconstriction (left), and nitroprusside (NTP)-induced vasodilation conditions. Variation of compliance in a single cardiac cycle, as well as the decrease of compliance with increasing pressure, are seen.

hypertension (mean pressure of 146±4.9 mmHg and 6.8 ± 0.2 mmHg/mL/s, respectively) compared to control (102 ± 5.3 mmHg, vs 3.4 ± 0.18 mmHg/mL/s, respectively). This result is expected, because methoxamine is a potent vasoconstrictor, primarily increasing peripheral resistance and BP. The characteristic impedance, $Z_o$, was not significantly affected. Pulsatile aortic blood pressue waveforms, and the corresponding instantaneous pressure-dependent compliances obtained at these three different conditions (Li and Zhu, 1994; Li et al., 1996) are shown in Fig. 7-9. Compliance, in general, decreases with increasing pressure. Vasoconstriction reduced arterial system compliance; nitroprusside-induced vasodilation greatly improved arterial compliance.

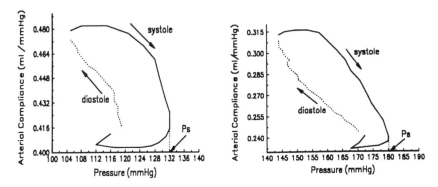

Fig. 7-10. The pressure-dependent arterial compliance plotted as a function of pressure for a complete cardiac cycle, or the compliance–pressure loop, at normal BP (left) and at high BP (right). Reduced compliance magnitude and compliance-pressure loop area are seen in hypertension.

The pressure-dependent arterial compliance plotted as a function of pressure for a complete cardiac cycle, or the compliance–pressure loop (Li, 1998), at normal blood pressures is illustrated in Fig. 7-10. Arterial system compliance maintains a value close to its maximum during this early ventricular ejection period, when aortic flow attains its maximum. Compliance begins to decline with continued increase in AoP and reduced aortic flow during the remainder of systole. At the end of the ejection, when aortic flow ceases, arterial system compliance is also at its minimum. In diastole, when aortic flow is zero, compliance follows an exponential relation, given by Eq. 7-5, increasing throughout the diastole toward maximum, readying for the following ventricular ejection.

At a higher pressure level, as in the case of induced acute hypertension (Fig. 7-10), the compliance–pressure loop has a steeper slope at early to mid-systole, indicating the compliance decrement is more dramatic with rising pressure and increased stiffness. Compliance, in general, is lower in magnitude, compared to control, for the entire cardiac cycle.

The dynamic changes in pulsatile pressure-flow relation are manifested as the compliance–pressure relation, which is fully encompassed in the dynamic compliance-pressure loop. Increased BP and decreased flow both serve to reduce arterial compliance. Conversely, a reduced arterial compliance serves to impede ventricular outflow and increase arterial pressure load. The reduced arterial compliance in the presence of other pressure-overloading structural alterations, such as aortic valve stenosis, can further deteriorate ventricular function (Li et al., 1997). The compliance–pressure loop concept, presented here, thus provides a new means for investigating the dynamic behavior of the arterial system under pulsatile flow conditions.

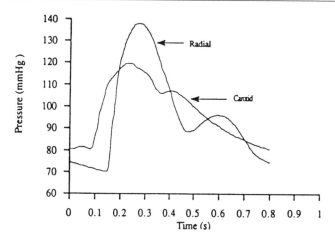

Fig. 7-11. Simultaneously measured carotid and radial pulses in a normal subject. Pressure amplification in the radial pulse and transit time delay can be seen.

### 7.1.4. PULSE WAVE VELOCITY IN HYPERTENSION

Increased PWV in hypertensive patients have been shown by numerous investigators and in many clinical settings (e.g., Nichols et al., 1993; Li et al., 1996). This is because PWV can be obtained noninvasively with tonometers or Doppler flow velocity probes. However, more detailed information can be obtained from apparent phase velocity spectrum. An example of simultaneously recorded BP waveforms in the carotid and radial artery of a normal subject is shown in Fig. 7-11. The peripheral amplification and the transit time delay of the onset of the pulse waveforms can easily be observed. Apparent propagation constant between these two sites can be calculated based on Eq. 4-22 shown in Chapter 4. The apparent propagation constant has been interpreted as pressure transfer function by some investigators. The apparent phase velocity calculated for this carotid-to-radial distance is shown in Fig. 7-12. At low frequencies, wave reflections dominate, and the resulting phase velocity is high, but, at high frequencies, there is increased damping, as well as out-of-phase cancellations of the propagating and reflected pulses: The phase velocity approaches the foot-to-foot velocity. With hypertension, the apparent phase velocity is greatly increased at low frequencies, as well as at high frequencies (Fig. 7-13).

### 7.1.5. PULSE WAVE REFLECTIONS IN HYPERTENSION

Increased systolic blood pressure and pulse pressure amplitude have both been attributed to increased wave reflections. Therefore, increased wave reflection has been suggested as a main contributor to systolic pressure augmentation. Indices such as reflection coefficient and augmenta-

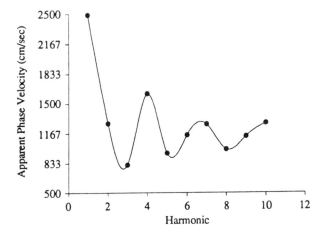

Fig. 7-12. Apparent PWV spectrum from carotid to radial artery distance for a normal subject.

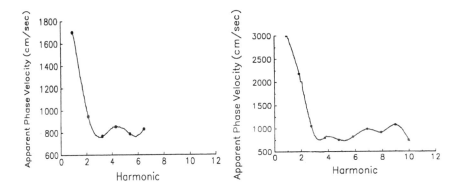

Fig. 7-13. Comparison of apparent PWV spectra for a normal (left) and a hypertensive patients.

tion index, have been shown to be significantly increased in hypertensive patients. These increases, as is shown in Subheading 4.4., are related to the vascular wall properties and the vasoactive states of the peripheral vascular beds. Therefore, there are structural changes associated with hypertension (e.g., Safar et al., 1984; Folkow, 1990).

The extent of hypertension associated changes differ in large and small vessels. This can be seen, e.g., in the simultaneously recorded ascending aortic and brachial pulses of a 54-yr-old man in control and 5 min after 0.3 mg sublingual nitroglycerine (O'Rourke et al.,1989), shown in Fig. 7-14. The pulse pressure is decreased in the aorta, but remains unchanged in the

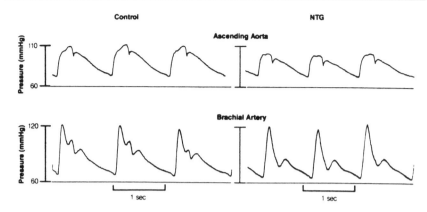

Fig. 7-14. Simultaneously recorded ascending aortic and brachial pulses in control and 5 min after 0.3 mg sublingual nitroglycerine. Notice that the PP is decreased in the aorta, and remains unchanged in the brachial artery during nitroglycerine, although the waveform morphology are both altered considerably. Adapted with permission from O'Rourke et al. (1989).

brachial artery during nitroglycerine, although the waveform morphology are both altered considerably. Vasodilators thus, alter the magnitude and timing of arrival of reflected waves. If one were to use the pulse pressure method (Stergiopoulos et al. 1994; PP is inversely proportional to compliance) to infer compliance changes, then there is little or no compliance change in the brachial artery during nitroglycerine. Because changes in wave reflection are always associated with changes in arterial compliance, the PP method may not be a good index of arterial compliance, apart from the aorta.

With hypertension, both the forward and reflected waves are altered, as demonstrated in Fig. 7-15. The commonly observed increase in PP and decrease in flow are obvious. The reflected pressure, $Pr$, significantly increased, and contributes to the systolic pressure augmentation in late systole. The forward wave, however, is also significantly increased, suggesting the response from the LV. The ratio of peak reflected wave to the peak forward wave differs from the augmentation index, defined by the ratio of augmented pressure over pulse pressure (Chapter 4). Notice that the times of occurrence of peak systolic pressure, and peak forward and peak reflected pressures, differ. Thus, their ratios can only be considered an empirical assessment. The reflection coefficient offers a better and more comprehensive assessment, although it is hindered by the use of Fourier analysis.

In hypertension, the heart works harder to eject against a greater arterial load: Whether this greatly increased power is beneficial for transmitting

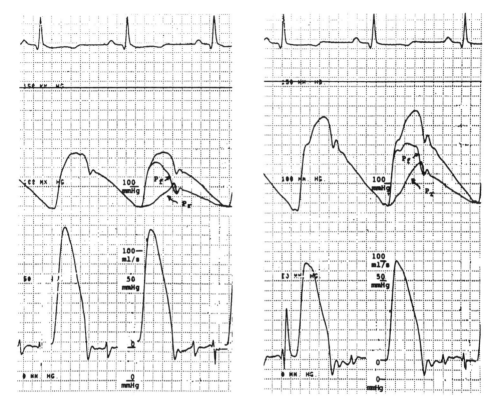

Fig. 7-15. Simultaneously measured ascending AoP and flow waveforms in a dog during control (left) and acute hypertension (right). Increased PP and decreased aortic flow are seen in hypertension. The reflected wave ($P_r$) is increased, causing late SP augmentation, but the forward wave ($P_f$) is also increased.

pulsatile energy to perfuse organ vascular beds has intrigued both researchers and clinicians. The amount of power generated by the ventricle and the amount that is transmitted to the peripheral vascular beds can be obtained from the consideration of forward and reflected waves (Li, 1989): This is illustrated in Fig. 7-16. The amount of power generated in hypertension and control calculated for the principal or fundamental harmonic associated with the forward and reflected waves are shown. The power generated in both cases is greater in hypertension than in control, but the net amount, or the power that is transmitted (the difference between the power associated with the forward and reflected components), is about the same. Therefore, in hypertension, a greater amount of power is generated by the heart, in an attempt to maintain adequate pulse transmission.

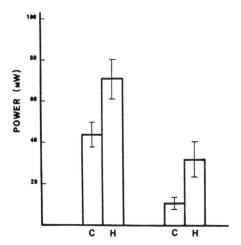

Fig. 7-16. The amount of power generated calculated for the principal or fundamental harmonic associated with the forward (left) and reflected (right) waves during hypertension (H) and control (C). Notice that the net amount of power transmitted (difference between the left and right) are about the same for control and hypertension.

## 7.2. Vascular Hemodynamics of Aging and Isolated Systolic Hypertension

### 7.2.1. FACTORS AFFECTING VASCULAR CHANGES IN AGING

Arterial blood pressure increases gradually with age. The change in systolic pressure is accelerated beyond age 55 yr, and the increase in pressure is greater for women than for men. The diastolic pressure, however, tends to level off; as is shown in Subheading 7.2.3., the increase in vascular stiffness or decrease in arterial compliance causes an increase in systolic pressure, and a decrease in diastolic pressure. The increase in mean blood pressure with slightly compromised stroke volume results in an increase in peripheral vascular resistance.

Blood pressure waveforms along the arterial tree change with age. Structure alterations of arterial wall properties, changes in the extent of vascular reactivity, and cardiac-related alterations are some of the contributing factors. As discussed in earlier chapters, the peripheral arteries are stiffer to begin with, therefore, increased vascular stiffness with age probably alters the more compliant vessels, such as the aorta and proximal large arteries, more than the smaller peripheral arteries. This is seen in Fig. 7-17, in which blood pressure waveforms from the ascending aorta to the femoral artery, at three different ages, are shown. With increasing age, the differences in central aorta and peripheral arterial pulse pressures become smaller. The increased SBP in aging is associated with both increased

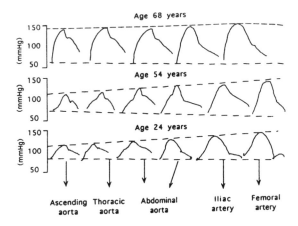

Fig. 7-17. Blood pressure waveforms along the arterial tree from the ascending aorta to the femoral artery, at three different ages. With increasing age, the difference in central aorta and peripheral arterial pulse pressures is smaller. Adapted with permission from Nichols et al. (1993).

PWV and increased wave reflections, as assessed by augmentation index (Fig. 7-18). The difference between the sexes is small in the latter.

Differences in morphological changes associated with aging are site-dependent, as shown in Fig. 7-17. These can be observed also in noninvasively obtained carotid and radial arterial pulses (Fig. 7-19; Kelly et al., 1989). The PP amplitude becomes larger, but smoother, suggesting increased arterial wall viscosity and viscous damping (Li et al., 1981; Wells et al., 1998) with age.

Increased pulse pressure and arterial load changes the coupling relation between the arterial system and the LV, as assessed by effective arterial elastance and ventricular end-systolic P-V relation (Chen et al., 1998), as shown in Figs. 7-20 and 7-21. Because both ventricular stiffness and vascular stiffness are increased, the coupling ratio of $E_a/E_{es}$ remains mostlyly unchanged. Parallel changes in cardiac and vascular properties have been observed also in chronic hypertension (Roman et al., 1996).

There are environmental and neurogenic factors associated with aging, which are, however, more difficult to quantify, unless well-designed longitudinal studies are carried out to investigate their mechanisms. An example of how living environment can affect vascular changes is shown in Fig. 7-22 , in which aortic pulse wave velocities are obtained from urban Beijing and rural Quanzhou residents of different age groups (Avolio et al., 1983,1985). The difference is striking. Stress-induced cardiovascular changes can be quantified (e.g., Pan et al., 1995), but the mechanisms underlying such changes have eluded many investigators.

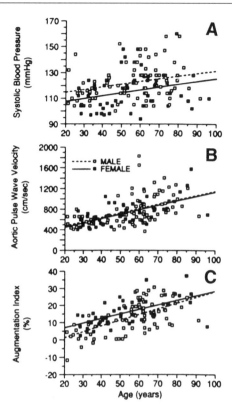

Fig. 7-18. Systolic pressure, PWV, and augmentation index increase with age. The differences in PWV and augmentation index are small between the sexes. Adapted with permission from Kelly et al. (1989).

### 7.2.2. ALLOMETRIC REPRESENTATIONS OF VASCULAR AGING

Allometric equations (Subheading 7.4.) established for the mammalian arterial system can be utilized to derive formulae for the calculation of arterial compliance and resistance at different ages.

For a man reaching adulthood at 20 yr of age, the corresponding compliance and resistance are calculated to be

$$C = 1.95 \text{ mL/mmHg} \qquad (7\text{-}8)$$

and

$$Rs = 1.15 \text{ mmHg/mL} \qquad (7\text{-}9)$$

The reduction in arterial compliance with age is more drastic than resistance, and can be approximated by an exponential relation, beginning at age 20 yr,

$$C = 1.95e^{-0.015(\text{Age}-20)} \qquad (7\text{-}10)$$

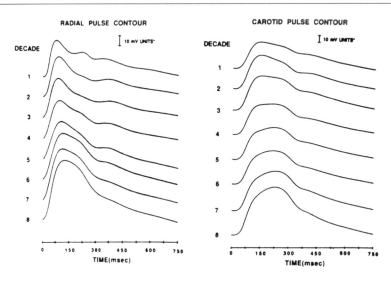

Fig. 7-19. Pressure waveform changes with age in the radial and carotoid arteries of normal human subjects. Adapted with permission from Kelly et al. (1989).

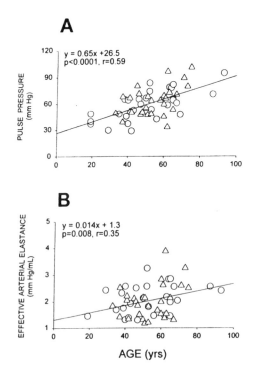

Fig. 7-20. Increases in PP and effective arterial elastance are observed with age. Adapted with permission from Chen et al. (1998).

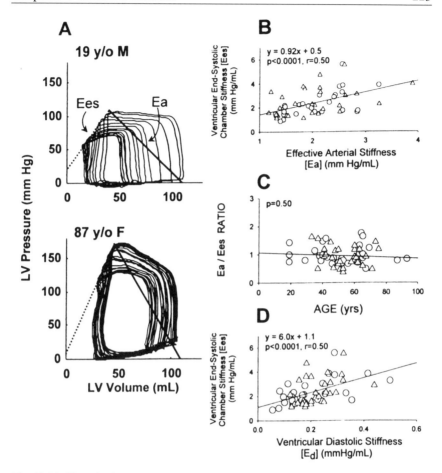

Fig. 7-21. Ventricular P-V diagrams for a young and an old adults showing both increased ventricular elastance ($E_{es}$) and arterial elastance ($E_a$) caused by increased stiffness. Their ratio ($E_a/E_{es}$) is mostly unchanged (*C*). Adapted with permission from Chen et al. (1998).

The increase in peripheral resistance is more gradual. Assuming such increase is linear, beginning at age 20 yr, we have

$$R_s = 1.15 + 0.008(\text{Age}-20) \tag{7-11}$$

From these two relations, it can be estimated (predicted) that, e.g., for a normal 55 yr-old man, the compliance is

$$C = 1.15 \text{ mL/mmHg} \tag{7-12}$$

about a 41% reduction in compliance, compared to the 20-yr old. The peripheral resistance is

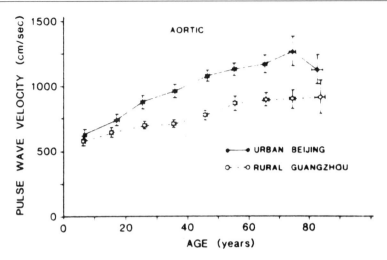

Fig. 7-22. Aortic pulse wave velocities obtained from urban Beijing and rural Quanzhou residents of different age groups. Large differences in adulthood are seen. Adapted with permission from Avolio et al. (1985).

$$R_s = 1.43 \text{ mmHg/mL} \qquad (7\text{-}13)$$

or an increase of 24% over the 35 yr. For a 70-yr-old man, the corresponding values are:

$$C = 0.92 \text{ mL/mmHg} \qquad (7\text{-}14)$$

and

$$R_s = 1.55 \text{ mmHg/mL} \qquad (7\text{-}15)$$

These represent a 53% reduction in arterial compliance and a concurrent 35% increase in peripheral resistance.

### 7.2.3. ISOLATED SYSTOLIC HYPERTENSION AND AGING

With aging, the vital organs of the body deteriorate in functions. Isolated systolic hypertension, is prevalent in the elderly (e.g., Safar, 1990; Frishman, 1991; Dart et al., 1993).). This is defined as a SBP greater than 160 mmHg and a normal DBP of 90 mmHg or less. We have shown that ISH is associated with a large (>75%) reduction in arterial compliance and a concurrently smaller (>25%) increase in peripheral resistance (Li and Berger, 1989; Berger and Li, 1990; Zhu, 1993; Li and Zhu, 1994; Li et al., 1994b). This was explained with the three-element windkessel model, which assumes that characteristic impedance is not significantly altered with aging and ISH, and that only $R_s$ and $C$ changes occur with advancing age and systolic hypertension. Thus, this model can be used to predict the gross features of the pressure waveform for any age.

Since aging adults (>55-yr-old) already have their arterial system properties modified to such an extent, as shown above in terms of vascular properties, the prevalence of ISH in this group is apparent. For instance, for a 55-yr-old an additional 35% reduction in compliance alone can lead to the production of ISH. This is even more so for the 70-yr-old, when only a little more than 20% decrease in compliance can make the 70-yr-old a candidate of ISH. Thus, vascular properties are considerably altered with the progression of normal aging.

The above model, because it is lumped, does not possess pulse wave propagation characteristics. In order to investigate the role of wave reflections in the production of ISH, we utilized the following relations, defined in Chapter 4:

$$P = P_f + P_r \tag{7-16}$$

$$Q = Q_f + Q_r \tag{7-17}$$

Pressure and flow waveforms can be resolved into their forward and reflected, or antegrade and retrograde, components. With the knowledge of the characteristic impedance in early ejection,

$$Z_o = (P - P_a)/Q \tag{7-18}$$

we can obtain the components as

$$P_f = (P + QZ_o)/2 \tag{7-19}$$

and

$$P_r = (P - QZ_o)/2 \tag{7-20}$$

Figure 7-23 illustrates the blood pressure waveform for a 30-yr-old subject with normal BP. Figure 7-24 shows the blood pressure waveform for a 60-yr-old normal adult. Figure 7-25 displays the typical ISH subject's blood pressure waveform. The difference between the last two is immediately apparent. With ISH, although the DBP remains normal, the SBP is substantially increased. As a result, PP is also significantly increased. This is associated with a significant reduction of arterial compliance and a slight increase in peripheral resistance, beyond normal aging.

In terms of wave reflections, comparing the normal 30-yr-old to the ISH subject, the latter has a significantly elevated reflected pressure component, although the forward component is also somewhat increased. The late systolic rise in reflected wave contributes to the substantially increased systolic pressure.

Figure 7-26 summarizes the observed waveform changes in terms of reflection coefficients for the normal young (30-yr-old), normal aging

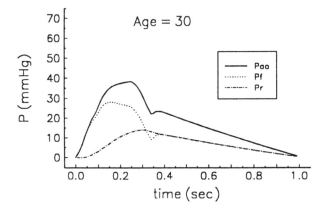

Fig. 7-23. Blood pressure waveform and the resolved forward ($P_f$) and reflected ($P_r$) components for a 30-yr-old subject with normal BP of 120/80. Only PP amplitude is shown.

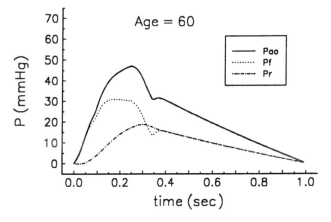

Fig. 7-24. Blood pressure waveform and the resolved forward ($P_f$) and reflected ($P_r$) components for a 60-yr-old subject with marginal normal BP. Only PP amplitude is shown.

(60-yr-old), and the ISH subjects. The ISH subject exhibits a consistently larger wave reflection for all harmonics. The differences are particularly pronounced at low and high frequencies.

Wave reflection could play a role in modifying pressure contour in ISH, as shown in Fig. 7-25 (Zhu and Li, 1995). Early wave reflections can augment systolic pressures in the aorta. The effect would be more pronounced in brachial artery, where conventional measurements are made. Thus, consideration of wave reflection may prove important if systolic pressure in ISH can be lowered by reduction in wave reflection, rather than by increasing arterial compliance through drug therapy.

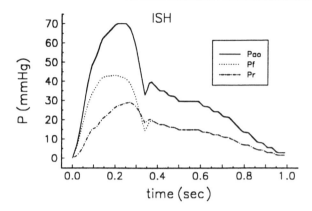

Fig. 7-25. Blood pressure waveform and the resolved forward $(P_f)$ and reflected $(P_r)$ components for an isolated hypertensive subject with BP of 160/85. Only PP amplitude is shown.

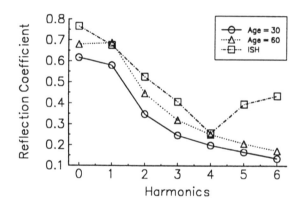

Fig. 7-26. BP waveform changes in terms of reflection coefficients for normal young (30-yr-old), normal aging (60-yr-old), and the ISH subjects. ISH subject exhibits a consistently larger wave reflections for all harmonics. The differences are particularly pronounced at low and high frequencies.

The use of normal flow waveform was based on published patient data. Simon et al. (1979) showed that elderly ISH patients and normals had similar heart rates (HRs), LV ejection times, cardiac indices, and ventricular ejections. Changing vascular properties in aging adults are a slow process in which the cardiovascular system of an aging person can adapt to the structural changes in arterial compliance and peripheral resistance over time, to maintain stroke volume.

Simon et al. (1979) showed that the only difference between older patients with and without ISH was that ISH patients had a decreased compliance. However, they also showed that there is a definite but slight increase in $R_s$. Adamopoulos et al. (1975) and Vardan et al. (1983) reported a sizable increase in $R_s$ in ISH patients. Normal aging has its effects on vascular properties, as well, so that peripheral resistance increases (James et al., 1995) and arterial stiffness increases, especially in the aorta, resulting in diminished compliance. Simon et al. showed that $R_s$ is higher in older subjects than in younger subjects. Thus, ISH is likely the result of an increase in peripheral resistance and a concurrent decrease in arterial compliance at levels greater than that normally seen in aging adults.

## 7.3. Aortic Valve Stenosis and Arterial System Afterload on Left Ventricular Hypertrophy

### 7.3.1. Double-Loaded Ventricle

Ventricular hypertrophy is an important adaptive mechanism that occurs in disorders associated with pressure or volume overload of the LV. Hypertrophy of the cardiac muscle is defined as an increase in the size of existing myocardial fibers (Panidis et al., 1984). The pressure-overload-induced hypertrophy, which is usually observed in valvular, subvalvular, or supravalvular aortic stenosis and in arterial hypertension, would cause concentric hypertrophy. In this case, the increase in LV mass is associated with a normal-sized LV internal cavity, and is characterized by an increase in the ventricular wall thickness-to-diameter ratio. The severity of aortic valve stenosis is assumed to reflect the degree of left ventricular hypertrophy, increased BP also compounds this process. There are many studies attempting to correlate the LV mass and wall thickness to blood pressure and/or the Gorlin-formula-derived valve area. However, because of associated confounding factors, the role that the arterial system plays when coexisting with aortic valve stenosis remains unclear. In this study, we developed an interactive model that affords examination of the individual effect of BP and aortic valve in the development of a hypertrophic ventricle, as well as the combined effects of coexisting aortic valve stenosis and hypertension, i.e., when a stenotic aortic valve and hypertension impose a double load on the LV.

### 7.3.2. Modeling and Analysis of Aortic Vave Stenosis

The left ventricle is geometrically modeled as an ellipsoid, as shown in Fig. 7-27, where $L_m$ represents the apex-to-base distance, $D_l$ represents the LV mid-wall chamber diameter, and $h$ the ventricular wall thickness. The LV volume ($V$) can thus be expressed as

$$V = (\pi/6) \times D_l^2 \times L_m \qquad (7\text{-}21)$$

The corresponding LV mass is

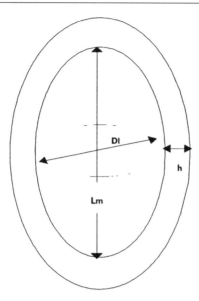

Fig. 7-27. Geometrical ellipsoidal model of LV, where $L_m$ represents the apex to base distance, $D_l$ the inner dimension, and $h$ the wall thickness.

$$LV_{mass} = 1.04 \times [\pi/6 \times (L_m + 2h) \times (D_l + 2h)^2 - V] \qquad (7\text{-}22)$$

where 1.04 is the mass:volume ratio.

The severity of aortic valve stenosis is represented in this model by the magnitude of aortic valve resistance, $R_v$ (Ford et al., 1990), which can be expressed as the pressure gradient across the valve over the corresponding flow,

$$R_{mean} = \frac{\Delta P_{mean}}{Q_{mean}} \qquad (7\text{-}23)$$

the pressure gradient ($\Delta P_{mean}$) across the valve can be calculated using Bernoulli's equation,

$$\Delta P_{mean} = (P_1 - P_2)_{mean} = \tfrac{1}{2}\rho(v_2^2 - v_1^2)_{mean} \qquad (7\text{-}24)$$

where $v_2$ and $v_1$ are flow velocity distal and above the stenotic valve, respectively. $R_v$ is calculated for the whole ejection period, and the mean value is used as the index for valve resistance. In the case of a normal valve with no evidence of stenosis, $R_v$ would be zero, indicating no pressure drop across the valve. The arterial system was studied using the three-element windkessel model, in which $R_s$ represents the total peripheral resistance of the arterial system, $C$ stands for the arterial compliance, and $Z_o$ is the characteristic impedance of the aorta. $P_a$ and $Q$ are aortic blood pressure and blood flow, respectively. Previous studies have shown that the hydrau-

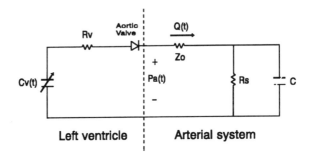

Fig. 7-28. Lumped-parameter model for the double-loaded LV, where $R_v$ is the aortic valve resistance, $C$ is arterial compliance, $Z_o$ is characteristic impedance, $P_a(t)$ is AoP, $R_s$ is total peripheral resistance, $Q(t)$ is aortic blood flow, and $C_v(t)$ is the time-varying LV compliance.

lic characteristics of the arterial system can be satisfactorily represented with a three-elements electric circuit (Subheading 3.1.). $R_s$, representing the steady-flow component of the system, can be calculated as the ratio of mean pressure to mean flow,

$$R_s = \overline{P}_d / \overline{Q} \tag{7-25}$$

and $C$, representing the pulsatile component, is calculated from diastolic aortic pressure decay from end-systole ($P_{es}$) to end-diastole ($P_d$), with $CR_s$ as the calculated time decay constant, $\tau$, where $t_d$ is the diastolic period,

$$P_d = P_{es} e^{-t_d / \tau} \tag{7-26}$$

The characteristic impedance $Z_o$ has generally been found to vary little in hypertensives, compared to normals, its contributing effect to LVH is assumed negligible in the current analysis. The lumped-parameter model for the double-loaded LV (Li et al., 1997) is shown in Fig. 7-28.

The wall stress of left ventricle can be expressed as the following,

$$s = \frac{P_{\mathrm{LV}} \times D_l}{4 \times h \times (1 + h/D_l)} \tag{7-27}$$

It is assumed that at increased afterload and/or the presence of aortic valve stenosis, at compensated hypertrophy, the increased LV pressure ($P_{lv}$) would cause the wall to thicken, to maintain a constant wall stress ($s$), while LV volume (V) and stroke volume are maintained constant. In this model-based study, increased LV pressure is the result of either a variation of $R_s$ and $C$ or an increase in $R_v$ only, or the combination of $R_s$, $C$, and $R_v$. Graded changes, at 10% steps in each parameter, were produced. LV wall thickness at compensated hypertrophy is thus calculated based on the constant LV volume and wall stress.

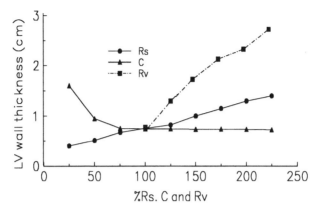

Fig. 7-29. Individual effects of changes in total peripheral resistance $(R_s)$, arterial compliance $(C)$, and valve resistance $(R_v)$ on LV wall-thickness parameter. 100% denotes normal value.

Figure 7-29 illustrates the individual effects of change in total peripheral resistance $(R_s)$, arterial compliance $(C)$, and valve resistance $(R_v)$ on the LV wall thickness parameter. From the model computation, an increase in either total peripheral resistance or valve resistance would lead to LV wall thickening. Changes in valve resistance, however, resulted in a larger hypertrophic response. Increases in arterial compliance beyond normal levels produced little alteration in LV wall thickness. A reduction in compliance to below normal level, as mostly seen in aging and hypertensive patients, resulted in an increase in wall thickness. Profound reduction of compliance by 75% would produce a significant increase in LV wall thickness.

Figure 7-30 shows the combined effect of concurrent changes in peripheral resistance and arterial compliance on left ventricular wall thickness. In this case a combination of increased peripheral resistance and decreased arterial compliance (as frequently observed in hypertensive patients), resulted in a greater increase in left ventricular wall thickness than either change in $R_s$ or $C$ alone.

In case of simultaneous increases in $R_s$ and $R_v$, as shown in Fig. 7-31 or when the heart is double-loaded with both increased afterload and stenotic valve, the process of wall thickening accelerates producing the largest increase in wall thickness.

Figure 7-32 shows the combined effects of changing arterial compliance and aortic valve resistance on the left ventricular wall thickness, which indicates that lowering arterial compliance would thicken the LV wall, and that increasing aortic valve resistance has a profound effect on the thickening process.

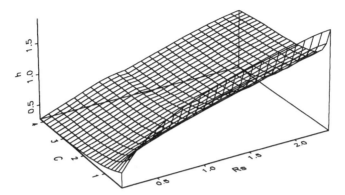

Fig. 7-30. Combined effects of changing both total peripheral resistance $(R_s)$ and compliance $(C)$ on LV wall thickness.

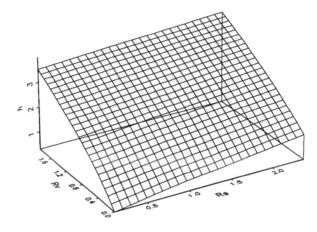

Fig. 7-31. Effects of changing both total peripheral resistance $(R_s)$ and aortic valve resistance $(R_v)$ on left ventricular wall thickness. Simultaneous increases in $R_s$ and $R_v$ on LV wall thickness.

Figure 7-33 graphically summarizes the individual and combined effects of hypertension and aortic valve stenosis on the development of left ventricular hypertrophy, which indicates that when aortic valve stenosis coexists with hypertension, the LV faces a greater overall load, and thus the process of hypertrophy accelerates.

### 7.3.3. RELATION OF AORTIC VALVE STENOSIS AND ARTERIAL LOAD IN VENTRICULAR HYPERTROPHY

Ventricular hypertrophy is an important risk factor for the development of heart failure, and is also an important adaptive mechanism that occurs

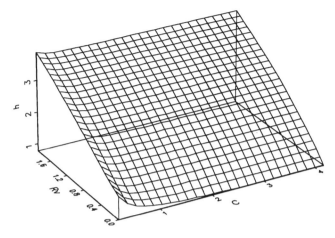

Fig. 7-32. Effects of changing both arterial compliance ($C$) and aortic valve resistance ($R_v$) on LV wall thickness.

in disorders associated with pressure or volume overload of the LV. Hypertrophy of the cardiac muscle is defined as an increase in the size of existing myocardial fibers (Ford et al., 1990). Consequently, it has been observed to be associated with an increased ventricular wall thickness. This growth process can be induced by a variety of physical and metabolic forces acting on the ventricle. The two main categories of hypertrophy are pressure-overload-induced hypertrophy and volume-overload-induced hypertrophy. Pressure-overload (as observed in valvular, subvalvular or supravalvular, aortic stenosis, and in arterial hypertension) would cause concentric hypertrophy, in which the increase in LV mass is associated with a normal-sized LV, defined as an increase in the ventricular wall thickness-to-diameter ratio. In pressure overload of the LV, the increase in wall thickness compensates for the increased systolic pressure and maintains a constant and normal LV wall stress, thus enabling the LV to eject a normal stroke volume against a high resistance. This mechanism can be best represented by Laplace's Law:

$$T = Pr/h \tag{7-28}$$

which states that LV wall stress is directly proportional to the LV pressure and chamber radius ($r$), and is inversely proportional to the ventricular wall thickness ($h$). With pressure overload, the wall-thickening tends to return wall stress toward normal. In a chronic compensated situation, this hypertrophic process is appropriate and compensatory (Li, 1986; Carabello et al., 1992). The constant wall stress assumed in the present model study is therefore justified.

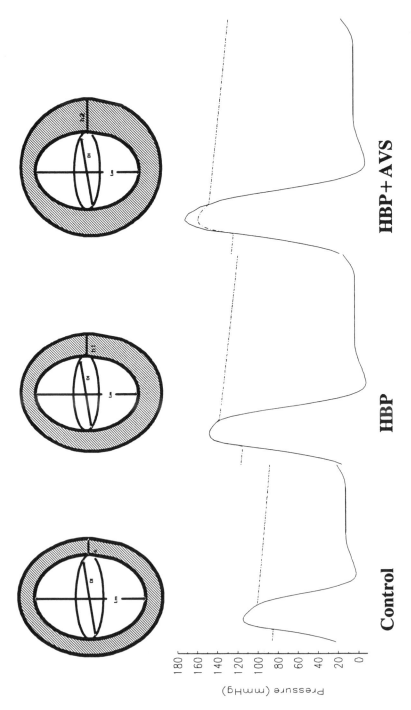

Fig. 7-33. Computer simulated data showing effects of hypertension (HBP) and aortic valve stenosis (AVS) on LVH. Upper panel shows model of LV and lower panel shows LV and AoP waveforms. A constant SV is assumed.

It has been observed that LV wall thickness and the degree of aortic valve calcification increase with the severity of aortic stenosis (Danielsen et al., 1991). Calcific deposits in the aortic valve are common in elderly patients, and may lead to valvular aortic stenosis (Aronow and Kronzon, 1991). Studies have shown strong correlation between pressure gradient across the stenotic valve and the LV wall thickness, yet only a weak relationship was found between Gorlin-formula-derived valve area and ventricular wall thickness (Schwartz et al., 1928; Reichek and Devereux, 1982). Thus, wall thickness alone is not a helpful indicator of severity of aortic stenosis, at least when aortic stenosis is quantified by the Gorlin-formula-derived valve area.

Even though hypertension would also induce LVH, only weak, though statistically significant associations were noted between LV mass index and both SBP and DBP (Mensah et al., 1993). This weak relationship can be explained by the fact that chronic overload is only one of several responsible factors, stenotic valve represents an important cofactor for the development of LVH. Systemic vascular resistance has a strong correlation with the severity of hypertrophy in hypertensive patients (Kimball et al., 1993). Even though myocytic hypertrophy and increased perimyocytic fibrosis accompany intraventricular pressure overload, as observed in both hypertension and aortic valve stenosis, studies have shown that there is an important difference between systemic hypertension and increased outflow resistance by valvular aortic stenosis, in that hypertension would cause intramyocardial arteriole wall-thickening and increased perivascular fibrosis (Schwartzkopff et al., 1992).

When arterial hypertension coexists with aortic valve stenosis, the hypertrophic heart faces two loads: valvular and vascular (noncompliant or stiff large arteries and constricted arterioles). Even though it is well known that both arterial hypertension and aortic valve stenosis induces pressure overload to the LV, the relationship between stenosis severity and systemic arterial hemodynamics is poorly understood. In particular, the influence of downstream events on proximal stenosis assessment is unknown. Arterial vascular load is an important determinant of LV performance (Li, 1987; Li and Zhu, 1994). Aortic valve stenosis cannot be considered as merely a valvular problem. On the contrary, it is a global problem relating to both the LV and the arterial system. With the ease of a well-controlled model (Zhu et al., 1994), we demonstrated the relationship between LVH and downstream load, as produced by varying valve resistance, total peripheral resistance and arterial compliance, corresponding to many clinical situations. In a preliminary clinical study, LV mass index, predicted by this model, correlated well with that obtained from echocardiography and carotid pulse (Ilercil et al., 1995). The incorporation of the importance aspects of the pressure-dependent characteristics of arterial system compliance (Li et al., 1990; Li, 1993; Li and Zhu, 1994) and pulse wave reflections (Li et al., 1996; Zhu, 1996) should further improve the usefulness of the model.

The interactive model presented above allows investigation of the interaction between the LV and the arterial system in hypertension, aortic valve stenosis and their combination. Changes attributed to aortic valve and the arterial system load parameters caused by varied severity of aortic valve stenosis resulting in increased LV wall thickness, can be quantified. Even though it is widely known that hypertension plays an important role in the development of LVH, the aggregating effect of hypertension on the development of LVH when coexisting with aortic valve stenosis has been unclear. The above model-based analysis shows that a coexisting stenotic valve and hypertension would augment the hypertrophic process with a greater increase in LV wall thickness.

## 7.4. Allometry and Its Diagnostic Applications

### 7.4.1. INTRODUCTION

The function and structural design features of the cardiovascular system have been considered to be optimal under normal physiological conditions. Structural changes have been suggested to adapt to functional demands, which requires substantial flexibility in adjusting the numerous control variables and set-points.

The complexity of the control aspects of the circulatory function has been unraveled only recently, but to a limited extent. The complexity arises from the constant physiological transformations needed for structural adaptation to meet functional demands. This complexity can be better appreciated from the beat-to-beat dynamic performance of the heart and its interaction with the vascular system. The complexity can be substantially reduced when appropriate scaling laws are imposed and relevant invariant features are identified.

In terms of structure and function, there are some characteristics that must vary with developmental stages and organ size, which are consequently scaled with respect to body mass, e.g., size of the heart, volume of blood, length of the aorta, and cardiac output. There are, however, characteristics that remain invariant, e.g., heart beats per life time, capillary, and red blood cell sizes. Many of these characteristics can be written as dimensionless numbers, and they reflect properties of the system that are difficult to change, because of constraints on the intrinsic properties of constituent biological materials.

Harvey, in his *De Mortu Cordis* (1628), made comparisons of the circulatory function from his many "Anatomical Exercises Concerning the

| The several Animals. | Quantities of Blood = to the Weight of the Animal in what Time. | How much in a Minute. | Weight of the Blood suf-tain'd by the left Ventricle contract-ing. | Num-ber of Pulfes in a Mi-nute. | Area of the tranf-verfe Sec-tion of de-fcending Aorta. | Area of the tranf. Sec-tion of af-cending Aorta. |
|---|---|---|---|---|---|---|
| | Minutes | Pounds | Pounds | | Square Inches | Square Inches |
| Man | 36.3 18.15 | 4.37 8.74 | 51.5 | 75 | | |
| Horfe 3d | 60 | 13.75 | 113.22 | 36 | 0.677 | 0.369 |
| Ox | 88 | 18.14 | | 38 | 0.912 | 0.85 Ri.   left |
| Sheep | 20 | 4.593 | 35.52 | 65 | 0.094 0.383 | 0.07 0.012 0.246 Ri.   left |
| Dog   1 | 11.9 | 434 | 33.61 | 97 | 0.106 | 0.041 0.034 |
|        2 | 6.48 | 3.7 | | | 0.102 | 0.031 0.009 |
|        3 | 7.8 | 2.3 | 19.8 | | 0.07 | 0.022 0.009 |
|        4 | 6.2 | 1.85 | 11.1 | | 0.061 | 0.015 0.007 |
| | | | | | 0.119 | 0.7 0.031 |
| | | | | | 0.125 | 0.062 0.031 |
|        7 | 6.56 | 4.19 | | | 0.109 | 0.053 0.032 |

Fig. 7-34. Some of the hemodynamic variables Hales quantified, including the blood pressure amplitudes and cardiac output in several mammalian species.

Motion of the Heart and Blood in Living Creatures," which he performed on several mammalian species, avians, and amphibians. Hales (1733) also performed these comparative experiments about a century later. Figure 7-34 illustrates some of the variables he quantified, including the BP amplitudes and cardiac output in several mammalian species. Interestingly, clinic assessment of circulatory function continues to consider BP and cardiac output as the most pertinent variables, even to this day.

Taking a different perspective, D'Arcy Thompson's *On Growth and Form* (1914) paved yet another path to modern comparative physiological studies by examining diverse collections of specimens. Looking at growth in relation to form, Huxley (1932) introduced the concept of differential growth to explain many observed biological transformations. He made clear that different organs and organisms may grow at differential rates in relation to body weight. Much of his interpretation was based on the use of allometric relations.

### 7.4.2. ALLOMETRY

Allometry is defined as the change of proportions with increase of size, both within a single species and between adults of related groups. The

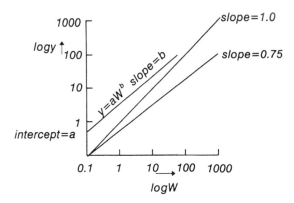

Fig. 7-35. Illustration of the allometric relations, with varying slopes according to the exponents of the power laws. $W$ = body weight.

allometric formula relates any measured physical quantity, $Y$, to body mass, $M$, with a and b as derived or measured empirical constants. Quantitatively, this results in a power law,

$$Y = a M^b \qquad (7\text{-}29)$$

This formula expresses simple allometry. In the special case when the exponent is 0, $Y$ is independent of body mass $M$. When b is one-third, or 0.33, then the variable is said to be dependent on body length dimensions; when b is two-thirds, or 0.67, $Y$ is dependent on body surface area, and when b = 1, $Y$ is simply proportional to body mass. This provides what is known as the basis of the one-third power law, or geometric scaling (Lambert and Teissier, 1927). This has recently been challenged by the one-fourth power law as the basis of biological allometric formulation (West et al., 1997). Figure 7-35 illustrates the simple power relations.

In the case of compound allometry, we have

$$Y = a M^b + c M^d \qquad (7\text{-}30)$$

The allometric equation has been proven to be powerful for characterization of similarities among species. It is effective in relating a physiological phenomenon, either structural or functional, among mammals of grossly different body mass. It can also be used for intraspecies comparisons. Allometric relations of some hemodynamic parameters are shown in Table 7-1.

A similarity criterion is established when $Y$, formulated in terms of either product(s) or ratio(s) of physically measurable variables, remains constant despite changes in body mass, and is dimensionless. Thus, the exponent b is necessarily zero. In other words, similarity is present when-

Table 7-1
Allometric Relations of Some Hemodynamic Parameters

| Parameter | Y | a | b |
|---|---|---|---|
| Heart rate (s$^{-1}$) | $f_h$ | 3.60 | -0.27 |
| Stroke volume (mL) | $V_s$ | 0.66 | 1.05 |
| Pulse velocity (cm/s) | c | 446.0 | 0.0 |
| Arterial pressure (dyn/cm$^2$) | p | $1.17 \times 10^5$ | 0.033 |
| Radius of aorta (cm) | r | 0.205 | 0.36 |
| Length of aorta (cm) | L | 17.5 | 0.31 |
| Metabolic rate (ergs/s) | MR | $3.41 \times 10^7$ | 0.734 |
| Heart weight (kg) | $M_h$ | 0.0066 | 0.98 |

$Y = a\,M^b$, M in kg.

ever any two dimensionally identical measurements occur in a constant ratio to each other. If such a ratio exists among different species, then a similarity criterion is established as the scaling law. This approach of establishing biological similarity criteria has been shown to be very useful (Stahl, 1963,1965; Gunther and Dela Barra 1966; MacMahon, 1973; Gunther, 1975; Li, 1987,1996).

### 7.4.3. BIOLOGICAL DIMENSIONAL ANALYSIS

Fourier (1882) emphasized the importance of dimensional homogeneity in making comparison of physical variables. Buckingham (1915), however, introduced the π- theorem of dimensional analysis, which states that, if a physical system can be properly described by a certain set of dimensional variables, it may also be described by a lesser number of dimensionless parameters that incorporate all the variables. This principle apparently was used to establish similarity rules at about the same time when Lord Rayleigh (1915) proposed the well-known Rayleigh indices, which can be illustrated by applying Laplace's law (Chapter 2) to mammalian hearts or blood vessels.

The formula for calculating force or tension has been based on the law of Laplace

$$T = p\,r \qquad (7\text{-}31)$$

which states that the pressure difference, $p$, across a curved membrane in a state of tension, is equal to the tension in the membrane, $T$, divided by its radius of curvature, $r$ (Woods, 1892). This law has been applied to both blood vessels (e.g., Burton, 1954) and the heart (Li, 1983). The equation indicates that a finite amount of tension in the wall is needed to balance the distending arterial pressure. Both arterial pressure and ventricular pressure are invariant in magnitude and in waveforms in many mammalian species (Fig. 7-36).

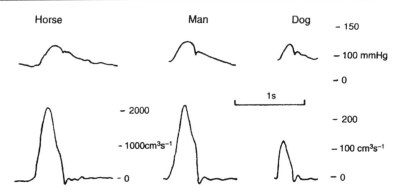

Fig. 7-36. Aortic pressure and flow waveforms recorded in different mammalian species.

In terms of the heart, we see that Laplace's law dictates that, the larger the size of the heart, the greater the tension exerted on the myocardium. To sustain this greater amount of tension, the wall must thicken proportionally with increasing radius of curvature. An increase in ventricular wall thickness is normally seen, which results in a larger heart weight or LV mass $(M_h)$. This modifies Laplace's law to the Lamé relation (Chapter 2),

$$T = p\ r/h \qquad (7\text{-}32)$$

It is clear that an increase in arterial blood pressure, as in the case of chronic hypertension, can also promote the increase in ventricular wall thickness, and hence cardiac hypertrophy.

A dimensional matrix can be readily formed by first expressing $T$, $r$, $p$, and $h$ in the mass $(M)$, length $(L)$, and time $(T)$ system. For instance, the radius has a physical unit of cm, in terms of [M, L, T] dimensions, it is [0, 1, 0], and pressure is force per unit area,

$$p = F/A \qquad (7\text{-}33)$$

and, since force is mass $\times$ gravitational acceleration

$$F = M\ a \qquad (7\text{-}34)$$

which has the dimension of gm cm/s/s, or $g^1$ $cm^1$ $s^{-2}$, or in terms of [M,L,T], it is [1,1,–2]. Area (in $cm^2$) has a dimension of [0,2,0], hence pressure has the dimension of [1,-1,–2].

The dimensional matrix for Laplace's law is then:

|   | $T$ | $r$ | $p$ | $h$ |
|---|-----|-----|-----|-----|
| M | 1   | 0   | 1   | 0   |
| L | 0   | 1   | –1  | 1   |
| T | –2  | 0   | –2  | 0   |

$$(7\text{-}35)$$

In order to derive dimensionless parameters ($\pi$), Buckingham's $\pi$-theorem is utilized. To reiterate, the number of $\pi$-numbers ($j$) is equal to the number of physical quantity considered ($n$) minus the rank ($r$) of the matrix (Li, 1983, 1986). Thus, there will be two $\pi$-numbers, $\pi_1$, and $\pi_2$.

$$\pi_1 = T/p\,h$$

and

$$\pi_2 = h/r \qquad (7\text{-}36)$$

They provide a description of the geometric and mechanical relations of mammalian hearts, and Laplace's law is implicit in the ratio of the two,

$$I = \pi_1/\pi_2 = T/p\,r \qquad (7\text{-}37)$$

### 7.4.4. INVARIANT NUMBERS AND DIAGNOSTIC APPLICATIONS

Both $\pi_1$ and $\pi_2$ and their ratio, $I$, are not only dimensionless, but they are also independent of mammalian body mass. That is, $\pi_2$ indicates that ratio of ventricular wall thickness to its radius, $h/r$, is invariant among mammals. This also establishes a scaling factor. They are thus considered invariant numbers, i.e., $[M]^0\,[L]^0\,[T]^0$ = dimensionless constant. This invariance implies that Laplace's law applies to all mammalian hearts (Martin et al., 1970; Li, 1986).

In the case of pathological cardiac hypertrophy, the h/r ratio is significantly altered as a consequence of increased wall thickness, which has been suggested as the result of an adaptation process by which the wall tension is normalized (Eq. 7-32). In a failing and enlarged heart, the greater tension caused by a larger radius of curvature results in excess myocardial oxygen demand. Cardiac size reduction via partial left ventriculectomy, or the Batista procedure, to normalize the h/r ratio and wall tension, has met with success in reversing this detriment.

Another example of scaling invariance can be found in blood flow in arteries. A dimensional matrix is first formed by incorporating parameters that are considered pertinent. These are the density ($\rho$) and viscosity ($\eta$) of the fluid, diameter ($D$) of the blood vessel, and velocities of the flowing blood ($v$) and of the pulse wave ($c$).

|   | $\rho$ ($g/cm^3$) | $c$ ($cm/s$) | $D$ ($cm$) | $\eta$ ($poise$) | $v$ ($cm/s$) |   |
|---|---|---|---|---|---|---|
| $M$ | 1 | 0 | 0 | 1 | 0 | |
| $L$ | −3 | 1 | 1 | −1 | 1 | (7-38) |
| $T$ | 0 | −1 | 0 | −1 | −1 | |
|   | $k_1$ | $k_2$ | $k_3$ | $k_4$ | $k_5$ | |

where $k_n$'s are Rayleigh indices referring to the exponents of the parameters. The $\pi$-numbers can readily be obtained. Two of these are the well-known Reynold's number, essential for identifying viscous similitude and laminar to turbulent flow transitions (Li, 1988), $R_e = \rho v D / \eta$, and the Mach number, $M_a = v/c$, or the ratio of blood velocity to PWV. Allometric relation gives

$$Ma = 0.04 \ M^{0.0} \tag{7-39}$$

which is invariant with respect to mammalian body mass. The Reynold's number is dimensionless, but is not an invariant function of mammalian body mass,

$$R_e = 260.76 \ M^{0.42} \tag{7-40}$$

Thus, dimensionless $\pi$-numbers do not equal similarity principles, i.e., scaling factors are not necessarily invariant numbers.

The different Reynolds numbers associated with blood flow in the circulation can be appreciated from in vivo blood flow measurement. High Reynolds number which exceed 2000, are often associated with flow turbulence.

### 7.4.5. ALLOMETRY OF THE CIRCULATORY SYSTEM

Allometric relations of anatomic structure and physiological functions are useful for identifying similarities of the circulatory function of different mammalian species (Li, 1996,1998). From a comparative physiological point of view, it is difficult to select the appropriate variables or parameters to describe precisely the circulatory function under a prescribed physiological condition. For this reason, circulatory allometric relations are generally obtained at resting heart rates (HRs). The obvious factors that are important in determining function are HR and size, cardiac efficiency and contractility, stroke volume and BP. Some examples of circulatory allometry are given in Table 7-1, and can be found in other sources (Juznic and Klensch, 1964; Stahl, 1963s 1963b,1965; Holt et al., 1968,1981; Calder, 1981,1996; Li, 1996,1998).

In mammals, the ratio of heart weight to body mass is an invariant, with the heart accounting for about 0.6% of body mass. In allometric form (Adolph, 1949; Gunther and DelaBarra, 1966), this is

$$M_h = 6.6 \times 10^{-3} \ M^{0.98} \tag{7-41}$$

where the heart weight, $M_h$, and $M$ are both in grams. With $M_h$ in g and $M$ in kg, this has been given (Holt et al., 1968) as

$$M_h = 2.61 \ M^{1.10} \tag{7-42}$$

It is readily apparent that experimental conditions and ecological factors can influence the empirical constants, a and b, as found in humans (e.g., Gugesell and Rembold, 1990; Lauer et al., 1994; Hense et al., 1998). The above exponents for the heart weight, however, do not differ significantly from the theoretical exponent of 1.0 ($M_h = M^{1.0}$). The deviations arise from statistical fits of regressions to experimental data. It is also readily apparent that, if a variable scales as $M^{1.0}$, then the allometric equation can be made invariant by taking a ratio with $M$ in denominator, i.e., normalizing with body mass.

The stroke volume ($V_s$) is also an invariant when normalized to heart weight or to body mass,

$$V_s = 0.66 \, M^{1.05} \text{ mL, or} = 0.74 \, M^{1.03} \text{ mL} \tag{7-43}$$

It has long been considered an important hemodynamic quantity in assessing ventricular function. Its product with BP, bears a direct relation to the energy expenditure of the heart, or the external work, $EW$,

$$EW = p \, V_s \tag{7-44}$$

This is the work performed by the heart to in order to perfuse the vasculature during each contraction, i.e., the work necessary to overcome the arterial load during each ejection. BPs are generally invariant with respect to body mass in mammals (of course, there are exceptions (McMahon and Bonner, 1983; Li, 1996), such as the giraffe (Goetz, 1960)). This also indicates that the heart is a pressure source, and that maintaining a constant BP is of utmost importance. The process of BP control is complex, and important roles are played by baroreceptors, the renin-angiotensin system, and the autonomic nervous system, just to name a few sub-systems. Allometrically, the mean AP is expressed as

$$p = 1.17 \, 10^5 \, M^{.033} \text{ dyn/cm}^2 = 87.8 \, M^{.033} \text{ mmHg} \tag{7-45}$$

The exponent is slightly, but not statistically significantly, different from 0 ($p = a \, M^0$).

Thus, the external work is given by

$$EW = 0.87 \times 10^5 M^{.063} \text{ ergs} = 0.0087 \, M^{1.03} \text{ J} \tag{7-46}$$

A larger ventricle generates a greater amount of external work. The quantity of blood that is ejected per beat (stroke volume), however, is a constant fraction of the amount contained in the heart (end-diastolic volume). Thus, ejection fraction, as it is termed, is an invariant among mammals,

$$EF = V_s/V_{ed} = 0.6 - 0.7 \tag{7-47}$$

In a failing heart, the ejection fraction can decrease substantially (e.g., to 0.2), as a result of a reduced stroke volume and an enlarged heart size.

The smaller the mammal, the smaller is its heart weight, but the faster its HR ($f_h$; Clark, 1927),

$$f_h = 4.02 \, M^{-0.25} \, s^{-1} \qquad (7\text{-}48)$$

Smaller mammals have shorter life-spans, since the total number of heartbeats in a mammal's lifetime is invariant. Within an individual mammal, rapid (and random) heart rhythms beyond normal often result in cardiac arrhythmias, such as ventricular tachycardia On the other hand, it is interesting to note here that "cardiac slowing," which reduces HR can actually have the beneficial consequence of increasing longitivity.

Cardiac output, deemed by Hales (1733) as an important quantity describing ventricular function, is given as the product of stroke volume and HR, or the amount of blood pumped out of the ventricle per minute,

$$CO = V_s f_h = (0.74 \, M^{1.03}) \, (4.02 \, M^{-0.25}) \, 60/1000 = 0.178 \, M^{0.78} \text{ L/min} \quad (7\text{-}49)$$

This is closely related to metabolic rate, since the heart supplies oxygen and nutrients for metabolism. Table 7-2 gives a comparison of cardiac output in several species. Deviations from this equation have been found in very small mammals (White et al., 1968). Because BP is invariant, cardiac output is limited by the total peripheral resistance to blood flow of the mammalian systemic arterial tree, which is obtained as

$$R_s = P/CO = 2.8 \times 10^6 \, M^{-0.747} \text{ dyn·s·cm}^{-5} \qquad (7\text{-}50)$$

Thus, the peripheral resistance follows the three-fourths power of mass (West et al., 1997), and is inversely proportional to the metabolic rate (+three-fourths). This relation can be strongly altered under local conditions, such as vasoconstriction or vasodilation. This derived allometric equation can be compared to that reported by Gunther and Guerra (1995) who gave an equation conforming more closely to the two-third power:

$$R_s = 3.35 \; 10^6 \, M^{-.68} \text{ dyn·s·cm}^{-5} \qquad (7\text{-}51)$$

### 7.4.6. THE ENERGETICS AND STROKE WORK OF THE HEART

The heart as a muscular pump, requires energy. The energy requirement of its constituent muscle fibers and the useful work it can generate are of considerable interest (Li, 1983a,1983b; Robard, 1959; Starling and Visscher, 1926). They define the mechanical efficiency of the cardiac pump. In hemodynamic terms, the efficiency of the heart is defined as the ratio of external mechanical work to myocardial oxygen consumption,

$$e = \frac{EW}{MVO_2} = Q_{cor} \times O_{2a-v} \qquad (7\text{-}52)$$

Table 7-2
Cardiac Output of Some Mammalian Hearts Based on
the Allometric Equation CO = 0.178 M$^{.78}$ L/min

| Species | BM (kg) | CO (L/min) |
|---|---|---|
| Elelphant | 2000 | 67 |
| Horse | 400 | 19 |
| Man | 70 | 5 |
| Dog | 20 | 1.8 |
| Rabbit | 3.5 | 0.5 |
| Mouse | 0.25 | 0.06 |
| Tree shrew | 0.005 | 0.003 |

BM = body mass; CO = cardiac output.

where $O_{2a-v}$ is the arterio-venous oxygen saturation and $Q_{cor}$, the coronary blood flow. The efficiency of the heart is an invariant among mammalian species (Li, 1996), and is about 20%. The relation dictates the energy requirement and pumping performance of the heart.

*EW*, also termed "stroke work," is represented as the area under the LV P-V diagram during each heartbeat. The external mechanical work generated by the heart per unit body, or heart weight, is constant for the mammalian species (Li, 1983a,1983b), i.e.,

$$\frac{EW}{M} = \text{constant} = \frac{pV_s}{M} \qquad (7\text{-}53)$$

This result is also of considerable physiological importance, since it states that the cardiac external work intensity, is invariant among mammals. Species differences in cardiac energetics, however, have been reported (Loiselle and Gibbs, 1979). For man, taking $V = 75$ mL, $p = 100$ mmHg, $M = 70$ kg, $M_h = 370$ g, the external work is about 1 J and the coefficient is about 2.7 J/Kg. In terms of heart weight, this is

$$EW = 2.7 \text{ J/kg or } EW = 1/70 \text{ J/kg} \qquad (7\text{-}54)$$

in terms of body mass. For a 2100-kg elephant, its LV is estimated to generate about 30 J for each heartbeat. Examination of the dimensions gives:

$$EW/M = [M]^0 [L]^2 [T]^{-2} \qquad (7\text{-}55)$$

which, although constant among mammals, is not dimensionless. Therefore, it is not an invariant number.

Cardiac output (Eq. 7-49) is a direct function of metabolic rate, following the three-qurter power,

Table 7-3
Physiological Parameters of Three Mammals Showing Relation of Metabolic Turnover
Rate to Heartrate

|  | Body mass $M$ (kg) | Metabolic rate $MR$ (J/s) | Metabolic turnover rate $MTR$ (J/s/kg) | Heart-rate $f_h$(1/s) | $MTR/f_h$ (J/kg) | $(EW/M)/(MTR/f_h)$ (dimensionless) |
|---|---|---|---|---|---|---|
| Man | 70 | 82 | 1.17 | 70 | 1.0 | 0.014 |
| Dog | 20 | 32 | 1.6 | 90 | 1.07 | 0.013 |
| Guinea pig | 0.7 | 2.6 | 3.7 | 240 | 0.93 | 0.015 |

$$CO \propto MR \propto M^{0.75} \tag{7-56}$$

Normalizing cardiac output or metabolic rate with respect to body mass gives

$$CO/M \propto M^{-0.25} \propto f_h \propto MTR \tag{7-57}$$

so that the metabolic turn-over rate (MTR) is a function of heart rate (Table 7-3). Combining Eq. 7-53 and 7-57 gives

$$\frac{EW/M}{MTR/f_h} = \text{constant} = K_h \tag{7-58}$$

The dimensions of $K_h$ are $[M]^0[L]^0[T]^0$ = dimensionless constant.

The value of $K_h$ is shown in Table 7-3. It is an invariant number, and serves to define the mammalian cardiac energetics in relation to the whole body metabolism.

### 7.4.7. VASCULAR PERFUSION AND ARTERIAL PULSE TRANSMISSION CHARACTERISTICS

The arterial system exhibits geometric and elastic nonuniformities. Geometric taper of the aorta is associated with increased elastic modulus away from the heart. Vascular branching occurs where target organ perfusion is necessary. Arterial wall thickness to lumen radius ratios are invariant at corresponding anatomic sites in mammalian species. Ratio of aortic length to diameter is also an invariant (Holt et al., 1968; Li, 1987). In addition, the sizes of terminal arterioles and capillaries, as well as red blood cells, are also virtually invariant among mammalian species, regardless of their body size. These represent structural invariants, giving rise to global vascular perfusion characteristics that are amazingly similar.

Similar pressure and flow waveforms are recorded in aortas of different mammalian species (Li, 1987,1996; Noordergraaf et al., 1979; Fig. 7-36). This suggests that corresponding pulse transmission characteristics may also be similar. Nonuniformities in geometry and elasticity, as well as viscous damping, give rise to varying impedances to blood flow along the arterial tree. Pressure and flow pulses are therefore modified as they travel away from the heart, as they encounter mismatching of these impedances. Impedance to pulsatile flow is like resistance to steady flow, and can be viewed as complex resistance that varies with frequency. Impedance is calculated as the complex ratio of pressure to flow for each harmonic, or multiples of HR. When the impedance is determined at the ascending aorta, or the entrance to the arterial tree, it is termed input impedance. Vascular input impedance ($Z_{in}$) can be used to characterize the global properties of the arterial system (Chapter 4).

When the characteristic impedance of the proximal aorta ($Z_o$) is matched to the input impedance of the arterial tree, i.e., $Z_{in}=Z_o$, maximum transmission is present, and reflection of the propagating pulse does not occur. Under this matched impedances condition, the pulsatile energy is totally transmitted to organ vascular beds. In normal physiological conditions, however, there is some mismatching of the impedances. This causes the reflection of the propagating pressure and flow pulses. The fraction of the propagating pulse that is reflected is given by the reflection coefficient, related to the impedances, as

$$\Gamma = \frac{Z_{in} - Z_o}{Z_{in} + Z_o} \tag{7-59}$$

The magnitude of the reflection coefficient at normal resting HR is about 0.4, which is similar for many mammalian species (Table 7-4).

Pulse propagation characteristics can be quantified with a propagation constant,

$$\gamma = \alpha + j\beta \tag{7-60}$$

where $\alpha$ is the attenuation coefficient, describing pulse damping due to viscous losses, and, $\beta$ is the phase constant, denoting the relative amount of phase shift or pulse transmission time delay caused by finite pulse propagation velocity, $c$. In the mammalian aorta, the PWV is invariant, as seen from the allometric relation

$$c = \omega/\beta = 446M^0 \text{cm/s} \tag{7-61}$$

where $\omega = 2\pi f_h$, $f_h$ = heart rate ($s^{-1}$).

To compare gross features of the arterial trees of different mammals, a modeling approach can be particularly useful. The lumped modified

Table 7-4

Data for Different Mammals for Analysis of Arterial Pulse Transmission Characterisitics

| | Body mass $M$ (kg) | Heart- rate $f_h$/min | Phase velocity $c(cm/s)$ | System length $l(cm)$ | Reflection coefficient $\Gamma$ | $\Gamma$ (expt) | Propagation constant $\times l$ $\gamma l$ |
|---|---|---|---|---|---|---|---|
| Horse | 400 | 36 | 400 | 110 | 0.36 | 0.42 | 1.13 |
| Human | 70 | 70 | 500 | 65 | 0.38 | 0.45 | 1.06 |
| Dog | 20 | 90 | 400 | 45 | 0.39 | 0.42 | 1.01 |
| Rabbit | 3 | 210 | 450 | 25 | 0.41 | 0.48 | 0.93 |

$Z_o/R_s = 0.1$ is used in the calculation of $\Gamma$ and $\gamma$.

windkessel model of the systemic arterial system has been shown to approximate the features of the input impedance of the systemic arterial tree. For this representation, the input impedance is

$$Z_{in} = Z_o + \frac{R_s}{1 + j\omega CR_s}$$  (7-62)

dominated by $Z_o$, $R_s$, and the systemic peripheral resistance as shown before.

It is clear that the peripheral resistance decreases and compliance increases with mammalian body size. Thus, the dynamic features of BP and flow pulse transmission can be scaled through this kind of modeling. The ratio of $Z_o/R_s$ corresponds to the ratio of pulsatile energy loss due to oscillatory flow to the energy dissipated due to steady flow (to overcome $R_s$), and has been reported to be between 5 and 10%, and is an invariant for the mammalian arterial circulation (Li, 1987,1996).

The total systemic arterial compliance, $C$, representing the elastic storage properties of the arteries is

$$C = 0.18 \ 10^{-4} \ M^{0.95} \ g^{-1} \cdot cm^4 \cdot s^2$$  (7-63)

Some of the pulse transmission characteristics for horse, human, dog, and rabbit are summarized in Table 7-4. The ratio of pulse propagation wavelength, $\lambda$, for the fundamental harmonic, to the length of the aorta, $l$, equals about 6, independent of the body mass of the mammal. The product of $\gamma l$ is about 1, again independent of the mammalian body mass and confirming that the propagation characteristics along mammalian aortas are similar. The global reflection coefficient is also practically invariant, despite vast differences in HR, systemic peripheral resistance, total systemic arterial compliance, and aortic characteristic impedance that are associated with different body sizes.

These observed phenomena concerning pulse transmission, PWV and input impedance, as discussed above, must all be attributed to a common mechanism. The architecture of the branching arterial junctions is such that only a portion of the pulse wave generated by the ventricle reaches the capillaries. Another part is reflected by the peripheral vessels, principally in the arteriolar beds. Reflected waves encounter mismatched branching sites on their return trip to the ventricle. As a result, a negligible fraction of the reflected pulse wave actually reaches the heart, with the exception of the fundamental frequency component, for which the wavelength is longer than the effective length of the vascular system.

Another important feature of the optimal design of the mammalian arterial tree network is that there is minimal loss of pulsatile energy due to vascular branching (Li et al., 1984). The vascular junctions are practically impedance-matched, i.e., the characteristic impedance of the mother vessel is closely matched to the branching daughter vessels. This implies that the geometric and elastic properties of the daughter vessels match that of the mother vessel. As such, pulse transmission at a vascular branching junction is met with minimal local reflection. This results in the facilitation of vascular perfusion with minimal energy loss en route to organ vascular beds.

### 7.4.8. THE OPTIMAL VASCULAR DESIGN CHARACTERISTICS

The cardiovascular systems of mammals exhibit amazing similarity in both structural and functional design characteristics. A larger mammal has a larger heart size, and is scaled with a greater number of fundamental building blocks: the sarcomeres, or muscle cell units. These sarcomeres change their lengths to provide tension for developing an invariant magnitude of BP necessary to propel blood to perfuse the vascular system. The cardiac efficiency and mechanical work intensity are both invariant features of the cardiac pump, and are only altered to meet changing vascular demands, such as activity. The mammalian cardiac energetics bears a constant relation to the whole-body metabolism, and this relation is maintained by changing HR to meet the demands of aerobic metabolism.

The geometrically tapered and branching design of the vascular system has nonuniform elastic properties. A larger mammal has a greater compliance of the aorta to accommodate a larger stroke volume. The peripheral resistance, is greater and closer to the heart as in smaller mammals, and is scaled to maintain an inverse relationship to cardiac output. Invariant pulse transmission features are embedded in the similar pulse pressure and flow waveforms observed at corresponding anatomical sites. The precision of natural design is even more amazing at vascular branching junctions, where branching vessel impedances are practically matched to ensure pulse wave transmission at utmost efficiency, with minimal wave reflection and energy losses.

The optimality of the natural design characteristics of the mammalian cardiovascular system are such that many features are preserved to be invariant across species, while similarities are governed by scaling laws.

## REFERENCES

Adamopoulos, P. N., Chrysanthakopoulis, S. G., Frolich, E. D Systolic hypertension: nonhomogeneous diseases. *Am. J. Cardiol.* 36:697–701, 1975.

Adolph, E. F. Quantitative relations in the physiological constitutions of mammals. *Science* 109:579, 1949.

Aronow, W. S. and Kronzon, I. Prevalence and severity of valvular aortic stenosis determined by doppler echocardiography and its association with echocardiographic and electrocardiographic left ventricular hypertrophy and physical signs of aortic stenosis in elderly patients. *Am. J. Cardiol.* 67:776–777, 1991.

Asmar, R. G., Pannier, B., Santoni, J., London, G. M., Levy, B. I., and Safar, M. E. Reversion of cardiac hypertrophy and reduced arterial compliance after converting enzyme inhibition in essential hypertension. *Circulation* 78:941–950, 1988.

Avolio, A. P., Chen, S. G., Wang, R. P., Zhang, C. L., Li, M. F., and O'Rourke, M. F. Effects of aging on changing arterial compliance and left ventricular load in a northern chinese urban community. *Circulation* 68:50–58, 1983.

Avolio, A. P., Fa, Q. D., Wei, Q. L., Yao, F. L., Huang, Z. D., Xing, L. F., and O'Rourke, M. F. Effects of aging on arterial distensibility in populations with high and low prevalence of hypertension: comparison between urban and rural communities in China. *Circulation* 71:202–210, 1985.

Bader, H. Dependence of wall stress in human thoracic aorta on age and pressure. *Circ. Res.* 20:354–361, 1967.

Berger, D. S. and Li, J. K.-J. Concurrent compliance reduction and increased peripheral resistance in the manifestation of isolated systolic hypertension. *Am. J. Cardiol.* 65:67–71, 1990.

Berger, D. S. and Li, J. K.-J. Temporal relationship between left ventricular and arterial system elastances. *IEEE Trans. Biomed. Eng.* BME-39:404–410, 1992.

Boutouyrie, P., Laurent, S., Benetos, A., et al. Opposing effects of ageing on distal and proximal large arteries in hypertensives. *J. Hypertens.* 10(S6):S87–91, 1992.

Buckingham, E. On physically similar systems; Ilustrations of the use of dimensional equations. *Phys. Rev.* 4:345, 1915.

Burton, A. C. Relation of structure to function of the tissues of walls of blood vessels. *Physiol. Rev.* 34:619–642, 1954.

Calder, W. A., III. *Size, Function and Life History*. Dover, New York, 1996.

Calder, W. A., III. Scaling of physiological processes in homeothermic animals. *Ann. Rev. Physiol*, 43:301, 1981.

Capello, A., Gnudi, G., and Lamberti, C. Identification of the three-element windkessel model incorporating a pressure-dependent compliance. *Ann. Biomed. Eng.* 23:164–177, 1995.

Carabello, B. A., Zile, M. R., Tanaka, R., Cooper, IV, G. Left ventricular hypertrophy due to volume overload verses pressure overload. *Am. J. Physiol.* 263:H1137–144, 1992.

Chen, C.-H., Nakayama, M., Nevo, E., Fetics, B. J., Maughan, W. L., and Kass, D. A. Couphing systolic-ventricular and vascular stiffening with age. J. Am. Coll. Coardiol. 32:1221–1227, 1998.

Clark, A. J. *Comparative Physiology of the Heart*. Macmillan, New York, 1927.

Corbo, M., Wang, P. R., Li, J. K.-J., and Chien, Y. W. Effect of propranolol on the myocardial contractility of normotensive and spontaneously hypertensive rabbits:

correlation of pharmacokinetics and pharmacodynamics. *J Biopharmac. Pharmacokinetics* 17:551–570, 1989.

Cox, R. H. Pressure dependence of the mechanical properties of arteries in vivo. *Am. J. Physiol.* 229:1371–1375, 1975.

Cox, R. H. and Pace, J. B. Pressure-flow relations in the vessels of the canine aortic arch. *Am. J. Physiol. 228:*1–10, 1975.

Danielsen, R., Nordrehaug,, J. E., and Vik-Mo, H. Clinical and haemodynamic features in relation to severity of aortic stenosis in adults. *Euro. Heart J.* 12:791–795, 1991.

Dart, A., Silagy, C., Dewar, E., Jennings, G., and Mc Neil, J. Aortic distensibility and left ventricular structure and function in isolated systolic hypertension. *Eur. Heart J.* 14:1465–1470, 1993.

De Bruyne, B., et al. Intracoronary pressure measurements with a 0.015-inch fluid filled angioplasty guide wire. In: Serruys, P. W., Foley, D. P., de Feyter, P. J., eds., *Quantitative Coronary Angiographiy in Clinical Practice*, Kluwer Academic, Norwell, MA, pp. 147–165, 1994.

De Bruyne, B. and Pijls, N. H. J. Coronary pressure measurements. *Primary Cardiol.* 21(5):29, 1995.

De Simone, G., Roman, M. J., Koren, M. J., Mensah, G. A., Ganau, A., and Devereux, S. R., Stroke volume/pulse pressure ration and cardiovascular risk in arterial hypertension. *Hypertension* 33:800–805, 1999.

De Simone, G., Devereux, R. B., Daniels, S. R., Koren, M. J., Meyer, R. A., and Laragh, J. H. Effects of growth on variability of left ventricular mass: assessment of allometric signals in adults and children and their capacity to predict cardiovascular risk. *J. Am. Coll. Cardiol.* 25:1056–1062, 1995.

De Simone, G., Daniels, S. R., Devereux, R. B., et al. Left ventricular mass and body size in normotensive children and adults: assessment of allometric relations and impact of overweight. *J. Am. Coll. Cardiol.* 20:1251–1260, 1992.

Devereux, R. B. and Roman, M. J. Inter-relationships between hypertension, left ventricular hypertrophyand coronary heart disease. *J. Hypertens.* 11:S3–S9, 1993.

Drzewiecki, G., Field, S., Mubarak, I., and Li, J. K.-J. Effect of vascular growth pattern on lumen area and compliance using a novel pressure-area model for collapsible vessels. *Am. J. Physiol. (Heart Circ. Physiol.)* 273:H2030–2043, 1997.

Folkow, B. Structural factor in primary and secondary hypertension. *Hypertension* 16:89–101, 1990.

Ford, L. E., Feldman, T., Chiu, Y. C., and Caroll, J. D. Hemodynamic resistance as a measure of functional impairment in aortic valvular stenosis. *Circ. Res.* 66:1–7, 1990.

Frishman, W. Epidemiology, pathophysiology, and management of isolated systolic hypertension in the elderly. *Am. J. Med.* 90(Suppl. 4B):14S–20S;1991

Frolich, E. D. Antihypertensive therapy: new concepts and agents. *Cardiology* 72:349–365, 1985.

Frolich, E. D., Sasaki, O., Chien, Y., et al. Changes in cardiovascular mass, left ventricular pumping ability and aortic distensibility after calcium antagonists in Wistar-Kyoto and spontaneously hypertensive rates. *J. Hypertension* 10:1369–1378, 1992.

Geipel, P. S. and Li, J. K.-J. Time and frequency domain identification of arterial system model parameters. *Proc. 16th NE Bioeng. Conf.,* pp.75–76, 1990.

Goetz, R. H., Warren, J. V., Gauer, O. H., Patterson Jr., J. L., Doyle, J. T., Keen, E. N., and McGregor, M. Circulation of the giraffe. *Circ. Res.* 8:1049–1058, 1960.

Gunther, B. Allometric ratios, invariant numbers and the theory of biological similarity. *Physiol. Rev.* 55:659, 1975.

Gunther, B. and DeLaBarra, L. Theories of biological similarities, non-dimensional parameters and invariant numbers. *Bull. Math. Biophys.* 28:9–102, 1966a.

Gunther, B. and DeLa Barra, L. Physiometry of the mammalian circulatory system. *Acta Physiol. Lat.-Am.,* 16:32, 1966b.

Gunther, B. and Guerra, B. Biological similarities. *Acta Physiol. Lat.-Am.* 5:169, 1955.

Gutgesell, H. P. and Rembold, C. M. Growth of the human heart relative to body surface area. *Am. J. Cardiol.* 65:662–668, 1990.

Hales, S. *Statical Essays Containing Haemostaticks.* London, 1733.

Harvey, W. *De Motu Cordis.* London, 1628. Dover ed., New York, 1995.

Hense, H.-W., Gneiting, B., Muscholl, M., Broeckel, U., Kuch, B., Doering, A., Riegger, G. A., and Schunkert, H. The association of body composition with left ventricular mass: impacts for indexation in adults. *J. Am. Coll. Cardiol.* 32:451–457, 1998.

Holt, J. P., Rhode, E. A., and Kines, H. Ventricular volumes and body weights in mammals. *Am. J. Physiol.* 215:704, 1968.

Holt, J. P., Rhode, E. A., Holt, W. W.,and Kines, H. Geometric similarity of aorta, venae cavae, and certain of their branches in mammals. *Am. J. Physiol.* 241:R100, 1981.

Huxley, J. S. *Problems of Relative Growth.* Methuen, London, 1932.

Iantorno, S. and Li, J. K.-J. Complaince indices in the assessment of cardiac diseass. *Proc. Internat. Conf. Eng. Med. Biol.,* 10:247–248, 1988.

Ilercil, A., Zhu, Y., Wu, J., Li, J. K.-J., Lee, M., and Nanna, M. Computer model prediction of left ventricular hypertrophy based on the concept of a double loaded ventricle. *J. Am. Soc. Echocardiograph.* 8:383, 1995.

James, M. A., Watt, P. A. C., Potter, J. F., Thurston, H., and Swales, J. D. Pulse pressure and resistance artery structure in the elderly. *Hypertension* 26:301–306, 1995.

Juznic, G. and Klensch, H. Vergleichende physiologische untersuchunger uber das verhalten der indices fur energieaufwand und leistung des herzens. *Arch. ges Physiol.* 280:3845, 1964.

Kelly R., Hayward, C., Avolio, A., and O'Rourke, M. Noninvasive determination of age-related changes in the human arterial pulse. *Circulation* 80:1652–1659, 1989.

Kelly, R. P., Gibbs, H. H., and O'Rourke, M. F. Nitogylcerin has more favorable effects on left ventricular afterload than apparent from measurement of pressure in a peripheral artery. *Eur. Heart J.* 11:138–144, 1990.

Kenner, T. Flow and pressure in arteries. In: Fung, Y. C., Perroue, N., Anliker, M., eds., *Biomechanics*, Prentice-Hall, Englewood Cliffs, NJ, 1972.

Kimball, T. R., Daniels, S. R., Loggie, J. M. H., Khoury, P., and Meyer, R. A. Relation of left ventricle mass, preload, afterload and contractility in pediatric patients with essential hypertension. *J. Am. Coll. Cardiol.* 21:997–1001, 1993.

Kleiber, M. Body size and metabolic rate. *Physiol. Rev.* 27: 511–541, 1947.

Klocke, F. J. Measurement of coronary flow reserve: defining pathophysiology versus making decisions about patient care. *Circulation* 76:1183–1189, 1987.

Lambert, R. and Teisser, G. Theorie de la similitude biologique. *Ann. Physiol. Physiocochem. Biol.* 3:212, 1927.

Lauer M. S., Anderson, K. M., Larson, M. G., and Levy, D. A new method for indexing left ventricular mass for differences in body size. *Am. J. Cardiol.* 74:487–491, 1994.

Levenson, J., Gariepy, J., Megnien, J. L., Merli, P., and Simon, A. Diuretics and arteriolar resistance and arterial compliance in human hypertension. *Eur. Heart. J.* 13(G):48–52. 1992.

Li, J. K.-J., McMahon, R., Singh, M., Zhu, Y., Amory, D., Drzewiecki, G., and O'Hara, D. Noninvasive pulse wave velocity and apparent phase velocity in normal and hypertensive subjects. *J. Cardiovas. Diag. Proc.* 13:31–36, 1996.

Li, J. K.-J., Zhu, Y., and Nanna, M. Computer modeling of the effects of aortic valve stenosis and arterial system afterload on left ventricular hypertrophy. *Comp. Biol. Med.* 27(6):477–485, 1997.

Li, J. K.-J. and Zhu, Y. Arterial compliance and its pressure dependence in hypertension and vasodilation. *Angiol. J. Vasc. Dis.* 45:113–117, 1994.

Li, J. K.-J., Cui, T., and Drzewiecki, G. A nonlinear model of the arterial system incorporating a pressure-dependent compliance. *IEEE Trans. Biomed. Eng.* BME-37:673–678, 1990.

Li, J. K.-J., Drzewiecki, G., and Wang, P. R. Compliance of the aorta in acute hypertension. *Proc. 7th Int. Conf. Cardiovasc. Syst. Dyn.* 7:1–3, 1986.

Li, J. K.-J., Zhu, Y., and Drzewiecki, G. Pulse pressure is a significant determinant of arterial compliance in hypertension and vasodilation. *Circulation* 90:I166, 1994.

Li, J. K.-J. *Arterial System Dynamics.* New York University Press, New York, 1987.

Li, J. K.-J. *Comparative Cardiovascular Dynamics of Mammals.* CRC Press, New York, 1996.

Li, J. K.-J., Melbin, J., Riffle, R. A., and Noordergraaf, A. Pulse wave propagation: *Circ. Res.* 49:442–452, 1981.

Li, J. K.-J. and Zhu, Y. Aging induced changes in arterial compliance and vascular resistance and its relation to systolic hypertension. *Am. J. Hypertension.* 7:87A, 1994b.

Li, J. K.-J., Zhu, Y., and Drzewieck, G. Arterial compliance changes in spontaneous hypertension and hypotension. *FASEB J.* A462, 1993a.

Li, J. K.-J., Zhu, Y., and Drzewieck. G. Difference in arterial compliance values measured at systolic, mean and diastolic blood pressure. *Am. J. Hypertension*, 6:41A, 1993b.

Li, J. K.-J. Increased arterial pulse wave reflections and pulsatile energy load in acute hypertension. *Angiol. J. Vasc. Dis.* 40:730–735, 1989.

Li, J. K.-J. Time domain resolution of forward and reflected waves in the aorta. *IEEE Trans. Biomed. Eng.* BME-33:783–785, 1986.

Li J. K-J. Comparative cardiac mechanics: Laplace's law. *J. Theor. Biol.,* 118:339–343, 1986.

Li, J. K.-J., Zhu, Y., and Drzewiecki, G. Systemic arterial compliance dependence on blood pressure: Global effects. *J. Cardiovasc. Diag. Proc.* 13:300, 1996.

Li, J. K.-J. Feedback effects in heart-arterial system interaction. In: I*nteractive Phenomena in the Cardiac System. Adv. Exptl. Med. Biol.*, 346:325–333, 1993.

Li, J. K.-J. A new similarity principle for cardiac energetics. *Bull. Math. Biol.,* 45, 1005–1011, 1983.

Li, J. K.-J. Hemodynamic significance of metabolic turnover rate. *J. Theor. Biol.*, 103, 333–338, 1983.

Li, J. K.-J., Melbin, J., and Noordergraaf, A. Directional disparity of pulse wave reflections in dog arteries. *Am. J. Physiol.* 247:H95–99, 1984.

Li, J. K.-J. Laminar and turbulent flow in the mammalian aorta: Reynolds number. *J. Theor. Biol.* 135:409–414, 1988.

Li, J. K.-J. and Berger, D. S. Concurrent compliance reduction and increased resistance in the manifestation of isolated systolic hypertension. *J. Am. Coll. Cardiol.* 13:244A, 1989.

Li, J. K.-J. A new approach to the analysis of cardiovascular function: Allometry. In: Drzewiecki, G. and Li, J. K.-J., eds., *Analysis and Assessment of Cardiovascular Function.* Springer-Verlag, New York, pp. 13–29, 1998.

Li, J. K.-J. and Noordergraaf, A. Similar pressure pulse propagation and reflection characteristics in aortas of mammals. *Am. J. Physiol.* 261:R519–521, 1991.

Li, J. K.-J. and Zhu, Y. Does increased pulse wave reflection contribute to isolated systolic hypertension? *Ann. Biomed. Eng.* 24:S-42, 1996b.

Li, J. K.-J. A new description of arterial function: The compliance-pressure loop. *Angiol. J. Vasc. Dis.* 49:543–548, 1998.

Liu, Z., Brin, K. P., and Yin, C. P. Estimations of total arterial compliance: an improved method and evaluation of current methods. *Am. J. Physiol.* 251:H588–H600, 1986.

Loiselle, D. S. and Gibbs, C. L. Species differences in cardiac energies. *Am. J. Physiol.* 490–498, 1979.

MacMahon, T. Size and shape in biology. *Science* 179:1201–1204, 1973.

Marcus, M. L. *The Coronary Circulation in Health and Disease.* McGraw-Hill, New York, p. 75, 1983.

Martin, R. R. and Haines, H. Application of laplace's law to mammalian hearts. *Comp. Biochem. Physiol.* 34:959, 1970.

McMahon, T. A. and Bonner, J. T. *On Size and Life.* Scientific American Library, New York, 1983.

Meister, J.-J., Tardy, Y., Stergiopulos, N., Hayoz, D., Brunner, H. R., and Etienne, J.-D. Noninvasive method for the assessment of nonlinear elastic properties and stress of forearm arteries in vivo. *J. Hypertension* 10(S16):S23–S26, 1992.

Mensah, G. A., Pappas, T. W., Koren, M. J., Ulin, R. I., Laragh, J. H., and Devereux, R. B. Comparison of classification of the severity of hypertension by blood pressure level and by world health organizatio criteria in the prediction of concurrent cardiac abnormalities and subsequent complications in essential hypertension. *J. Hypertens.* V11:1429–1440, 1993.

Merillon, J. P., Fontenier, G. J., Lerallut, J. F., and Jaffrin, M. Y. Aortic input impedance in normal man and arterial hypertension: Its modification during changes in aortic pressure. *Cardiovasc. Res.* 16:646-656;1982

Milio, G., Cospite, V., and Cospite, M. Hypertension and peripheral arterial disease: a plethysmographic study. *Angiol. J. Vasc. Dis.* 48:241–245, 1997.

Nichols, W. M., O'Rourke, M. F., Avolio, A. P., Yaginuma, T., Murgo, J. P., Pepine, C. J., and Conti, C. R. Effects of age on ventricular-vascular coupling. *Am. J. Cardiol.* 55:1179–1184;1985

Nichols, W. W. and McDonald, D. A. Wavevelocity in the proximal aorta. *Med. Biol. Eng.* 10: 327–335, 1972.

Nichols, W.W., A.P. Avolio, R.P. Kelly et al. Effects of age and of hypertension on wave travel and reflections. In: O'Rourke, M. F., Safar, M., and Dzau, V., eds., *Arterial Vasodilation: Mechanisms and Therapy.* Edward Arnold, London, pp. 23–40, 1993.

Noordergraaf, A., Li, J. K.-J., and Campbell, K. B. Mammalian hemodynamics: a new similarity principle. *J. Theor. Biol.*, 79:485, 1979.

Opie, L. H. *Drugs for the Heart.* W.B. Saunders, Philadelphia, 1995.

O'Rourke, M. F. and Taylor, M. G. Vascular impedance of the femoral bed. *Circ. Res.* 18:126–139, 1966.

O'Rourke, M. F., Kelly, R. P., Avolio, A. P., et al. Effects of arterial dilator agents on central aortic systolic pressure and on left ventricular hydraulic load. *Am. J. Cardiol.* 63:38I–44I, 1989.

Pan, R. L.-C., Li, J. K.-J., Zhu, Y., and Drzewiecki, G. Noninvasive continuous measurement of autonomic function during Valsalva manuver: use for hypertension evaluation. *Am. J. Hypertnsion* 8:62A, 1995.

Panidis, J. P., Kotler, M. N., Ren, J. F., Mintz, G. S., Ross, J., and Kalman, P. Development and regression of left ventricular hypertrophy. *J. Am. Coll. Cardiol.* 3(5):1309–1320, 1984.

Peterson, L. H., Jensen, R. E., and Parrel, J. Material properties of arteries in vivo. *Circ. Res.* 8:622–639, 1960.

Pickering, T. G. Hypertension: definitions, natural histories and consequences. *Am. J. Med.* 52:570–583, 1972.

Pickering, G. W. *High Blood Pressure.* Churchill, London, 1955.

Pickering, G. W. The peripheral resistance in persistent arterial hypertension. *Clin. Sci.* 2:209, 1936.

Randall, O. S., VanDenBos, G. C., and Westerhof, N. Systemic compliance: Does it play a role in the genesis of essential hypertension? *Cardiovasc. Res.* 18:455–462, 1984.

Reichek, N. and Devereux, R. B. Reliable estimation of peak left ventricular systolic pressure by M-mode echocardiographic-determined end-diastolic relative wall thickness. *Am. Heart J.* 103:202–209, 1982.

Robard, S., Williams, F., and Williams, C. The spherical dynamics of the heart. *Am. Heart J.* 57:348–360, 1959.

Roman, M. J., Pickering, T. G., Schwartz, J. E., Pini, R., and Devereux, R. B. Relation of arteial structure and function to left ventricular geometric patterns in hypertensive adults. *J. Am. Coll. Cardiol.* 28:751–756, 1996.

Roman, M. J., Pini, R., Pickering, T. G., and Devereux, B. Noninvasive measurements of arterial compliance in hypertensive compared with normotensive adults. *J. Hypertension* 10(6):S115–S118, 1992.

Safar, M. Aging and its effects on the cardiovascular system. *Drugs* 39(Suppl. 1):1–8, 1990.

Safar ME, Simon AC, Levenson JA: Structural changes of large arteries in sustained essential hypertension. *Hypertension* 6(SIII): 117–121, 1984.

Schwartz, A., Vignola, P. A., Kalker, H. J., King, M. E., and Goldblatt, A. Echocardiographic estimation of aortic valve gradient in aortic stenosis. *Ann. Intern. Med.* 89:329–335, 1978.

Schwartzkopff, R., Frenzel, H., Dieckerhoff, J., Betz, P., Flasshove, M., Schulte H. D., et al. Morphometric investigation of human myocardium in arterial hypertension and valvular aortic stenosis. *Eur. Heart J.* 13(Suppl D):17–23, 1992.

Simon, A. C., Levenson, J. A., Chau, N. P., and Pithois-Merli, I. Role of arterial compliance in the physiopharmacological approach to human hypertension. *J. Cardiovasc. Pharmacol.* 19(S5):11–20, 1992.

Simon, A. C., Safar, M. E., Levenson JA, London GM, Levy BI, Chau NP: An evaluation of large arteries compliance in man. *Am. J. Physiol.* 237:H550–554, 1979.

Stahl, W. R. Organ weights in primates and other mammals. *Science* 150:1039–1042, 1965.

Stahl, W. R. Similarity analysis of biological systems. *Persp. Biol. Med.* 6:291, 1963.

Stahl, W.R. The analysis of biological similarity. *Adv. Biol. Med. Phys.*, 9:356, 1963.

Starling, E. H. and. Visscher, M. B. The regulation of the energy output of the heart. *J. Physiol.* 62:243–261, 1926.

Stergiopoules, N., Meister, J. J., and Westerhof, N. Simple and accurate way for estimating total and segmental compliance. *Ann. Biomed. Eng.* 22:392–397, 1994.

Thompson, D. W. *On Growth and Form.* Cambridge University Press, Cambridge, UK, 1917.

Ting, C., Yang, T., Chen, J., Chen, M., and Yin, F. C. P. Arterial hemodynamics in human hypertension. Effects of angiotensin converting enzyme inhibitors. *Hypertension* 22:839–846, 1993.

Trazzi, S., Ravogli, A., Villani, A., Santucciu, C., Giannattasio, C., Cattaneo, B. M., and Mancia, G. Early cardiac and vascular structural changes in subjects with parental hypertension. *J. Hypertension.* 11(S5):78–S79, 1993.

Vardan, S., Mookherjee, S., Warner, R., and Smulyan, H. Systolic hypertension in the elderly: Hemodynamic response to long-term thiazide diuretic therapy and its side effects. *JAMA* 250:2807–2813;1983

Wells, S. M., Langille, B. L., and Adamson, S. L. In vivo and in vitro mechanical properties of the sheep in thoracic aorta and in the perinatal period and adulthood. *Am. J. Physiol.* 274:H1749–H1760, 1998.

West, G. B., Brown, J. H., and Enquist, B. J. A general model for the origin of allometric scaling laws in biology. *Science* 276:122–126, 1997.

Westling H., Jansson, L., Johnson, B., et al. Vasoactive drugs and elastic properties of human arteries in vivo, withj special reference to the action of nitroglycerine. *Eur. Heart J.* 5:609–616, 1984.

White, L., Haines, H., and Adams, T. Cardiac output related to body weights in small mammals. *Comp. Biochem. Physiol.* 27:559–565, 1968.

Woods, R. H. A few applications of a physical theorem to membranes in the human body in a state of tension. *J. Anat. Physiol.* 26:362–370, 1892.

Zakzewski, C., Li, J. K.-J., Amory, D., and Jaisaitis, D. Iontophoretically enhanced transdermal drug delivery of an angiotensin-converting enzyme inhibitor in induced hypertensive rabbits. *Cardiovas. Drugs Ther.* 6:589–596, 1992.

Zhu, Y., Nanna ,M., and Li, J. K.-J. Effects of combined arterial system load and aortic valve stenosis on left ventricular hypertrophy: A model based study. *J. Cardiovasc. Diag. Proc.* 12:115, 1994.

Zhu, Y. *Computer Based Analysis of Systolic/Diastolic Left Ventricular Function and Pressure-Dependent Arterial Compliance.* Ph.D. dissertation, Rutgers University, NJ, 1996.

Zhu, Y. *Hemodynamic Basis And Nonlinear Model Analysis of Hypertension and Aging.* MS Thesis, Rutgers University. 1993.

Zhu, Y., Dai, J. W., and Li, J. K.-J. Total systemic arterial compliance: evaluation of time and frequency domain methods. *Proc. 21st NE Bioeng. Conf.*, pp. 4–6, 1995.

Zhu, Y. and Li, J. K.-J. Isolated systolic hypertension:the role of systolic wave reflections. *Am. J. Hypertension* 8:62A, 1995.

# INDEX

From: *The Arterial Circulation: Physical Principles and Clinical Applications*
By: J. K-J. Li © Humana Press Inc., Totowa, NJ